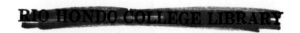

POPULATION CONTROL: FOR & AGAINST

POPULATION CONTROL: FOR & AGAINST

INTRODUCTION BY HAROLD H. HART

Hart Publishing Company, Inc.
New York City

Contents

Introduction

When the Aswan Dam was being built, economists and agriculturists optimistically anticipated that the resultant improved irrigation would dramatically increase Egypt's food supply. And while the enthusiasm for the dam was at its height, other more pessimistic economists and demographers pointed out that by the time the dam was completed, children would have been born in Egypt in sufficient numbers to more than consume the additional food supply. The dam would not ameliorate Egypt's lack of food.

For many countries, population control is the prime —in fact, the only—solution for the major problems which beset these underdeveloped economies. But the dismaying fact is that population control is more difficult to achieve in the places where it is sorely needed than in the countries where the economy can support its population. Witness in this regard the United States, which during the past few years, without the imposition of official controls, has achieved approximately a zero population growth. A key concern then is how population control can be achieved in countries where illiteracy is high, where communication is difficult, and where custom and religion conspire to thwart education in this regard.

The writers who have contributed to this volume

agree that to be effective any system of population control would involve a severe curtailment of personal liberty. In fact, some consider that it might be a totally unacceptable curtailment of personal liberty. For many of the essayists, the means necessary to achieve the desideratum might be too heinous to justify the needed procedures.

This moral and philosophical question is one which you, the reader, will settle for yourself after reading the pros and cons set forth in this provocative volume. If there are five men in a boat which must sink unless one man is thrown overboard, is there an acceptable way to sacrifice the life of one in order to save the other four? Is it immoral and unacceptable to legally and forcibly prohibit people from bearing children although the inevitable result of unchecked population growth is that all people in the community will be irretrievably harmed?

There are many "ifs" in this last paragraph. These significant issues are the subject of this challenging book.

HAROLD H. HART

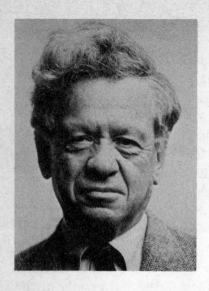

Max Lerner, author, teacher and journalist, is currently professor of American Civilization and World Politics at Brandeis University. As a journalist and scholar, he has traveled to almost every part of the world, and has lectured before university groups on six continents.

His newspaper column, which he writes three times a week, appears in the NEW YORK POST, *and is widely syndicated both in the United States and internationally.*

Mr. Lerner has written a dozen books, of which the best known is AMERICA AS A CIVILIZATION. *His most recently published book is* TOCQUEVILLE AND AMERICAN CIVILIZATION.

Max Lerner

Count me as one who believes the population growth must be slackened, checked, and in the end kept carefully in balance with the other major elements of the total ecological system. As a possibilist, I know it can be done for America and the developed societies—provided the collective will is there to do it. I am less certain that the will can be found for many of the developing societies, who feel their major problem is to stimulate economic growth and who can't think about striking a balance until they have done so.

We are entering a third period in the history of population control. The first was the Malthusian, based on the idea of a balance in nature between population increase and the food supply. There were curious sexual overtones in the thinking of Malthus (the leading parson in what Marx called the "hour of the parsons"), as he invoked the damnation of floods, famines, pestilences, and other acts of God for the sin of giving way to the sexual and propagative drives. But there was also a belief in the capacity to reform society by acting on the birth rate, which the population control movement has never lost.

The second period, the neo-Malthusian, drew the remedy implicit in the Malthus essay, which he had himself been too inhibited to draw. For while he was a man of commanding stature, and was attacked by the bluenoses of the day for daring to write about birth quantitatively, he also cared deeply about "virtue and purity of manners," and about "virtuous love, exalted by friendship" as the only basis of sexuality. He considered such social and sexual reformers as Condorcet and Godwin to be little better than libertines. In Chapter 8 of his famous essay, he taxes the Frenchman with speaking of "a promiscuous concubinage, which would prevent breeding, or do something else as unnatural"—presumably the condom. Thus, what came to be known by his name, as neo-Malthusianism, would have thrown a scare into the good clergyman.

The movement was part of a heroic age with heroes and heroines all the way from Francis Place—the London haberdasher and labor organizer who in the early nineteenth century printed a four-page pocket pamphlet, "To the Married of Both Sexes of the Working People," telling them how they could "do as other people do, to avoid having more children than they wish to have"—through Annie Besant, Charles Bradlaugh, and Margaret Sanger, to the handful of devoted contemporaries today who have risked dangers and laid their careers on the line in order to get open discussion and acceptance of the anti-natal technology (birth control, abortion, sterilization).

No brilliant intellectual feat like that of Malthus was required in this phase of the movement, whose invested talents were mainly of technology, publicity, education—

along with the willingness to risk martyrdom in the form of jail sentences and social obloquy. The underlying philosophy of this phase was that the social and legal acceptance of a birth-control technology would give each family the chance to plan its own destiny in terms of natality, would avoid the added governmental and social costs of unwanted children, would fortify the mental health of parents and children alike, would give the woman a better chance to fulfill her potentials, and would add to the strength of the marriage ties rather than break them.

The second phase achieved a breakthrough in America in the nineteen-sixties. It is still in effect, but no longer as a martyr-and-hero movement nor one needing publicity. One thing that has happened to it, as it has turned and enlarged into the third phase, is that it has become a triumphant, almost swaggering movement, feeding and being fed by the total sexual revolution and the woman's revolution. The whole mood and climate of the time have changed. In the old days, before The Flood, the myth was that you didn't dare say anything against American motherhood. Today you not only can but you do. In any anti-natal group the courageous thing is to say anything *for* motherhood.

Almost the whole of the neo-Malthusian movement for birth control was conducted in a climate of puritanism, of Victorian morals. It was this Victorianism that made possible the antics of Anthony Comstock and the New York Society for the Suppression of Vice, throwing hundreds into jail and spreading terror among the natal reformers, before he became a laughingstock for his excesses. But the censorship over books, pamphlets, and the rest was far less important than the built-in taboos most people felt against discussing contraception or abortion, or even using the terms. It was the internalized recoil that counted, and until that could be overcome the prospects of effective population control were scanty.

The taboos are scarcely visible any more. They were overcome by successive sexual revolutions, in almost every decade from the twenties through the sixties. Population control as a policy movement couldn't have come through unless the path had been cleared by the attitude revolutions, not only in the use of contraceptive technology but in sexual knowledge, sexual attitudes, and the heightened consciousness of women as women.

Let me say a word here about the rhetoric of a social movement but also about its logic, for both are important. The rhetoric gives it a propulsive force; the logic hems it in, steadies it, makes it zero in on its true target. The rhetoric of Malthusianism was a mathematical rigor of historic and natural law that depressed the few and left the many feeling helpless. The rhetoric of neo-Malthusianism was freedom—the freedom of the mates to play their own fate by choosing how many children they would or would not have. For a time Margaret Sanger, who first used the honest term "birth control," frightened off many of the potential faithful by raising the specter of control, and thus parading the wrong rhetoric. Then the public-relations mind got around to the semantic problem, and lo and behold, the term became "family planning," with the emphasis on the freedom of parents to plan their lives according to their best lights—and there we were, back in the rhetoric of freedom, and have been ever since.

I am not carping nor being nasty, and I trust I am not simplifying. The traditional movement has been part of a great complex of urgencies—for better fertility research, for better contraceptive technology, for establishing free clinics, for abortion reform, for sex education in the schools (including the medical schools), for the education of churches and churchmen, for a healthy climate of opinion that will cope with religious and other barriers to birth control, with pressure on legislatures, and with the whole legislative span of anti-natalist measures.

The cause is an appealing one. It is to make life more tolerable for mothers and their families by making freedom of natal choice a reality for them. It is—by preventing the unwanted children from being born—to give the wanted ones a better chance at life's chances. It is to help developing countries to a toehold in the age-long wrestling with the problem of too many mouths for too little food. In the developed countries, it is to give some outer breathing-space to the congested cities, and some inner breathing-space to the family, and especially the woman. Never have so many been served so well by the efforts of a relative few.

But a nagging question persists. Freedom of choice is a thrilling watchword to blazon on the banners of the movement, to raise a standard that young and old, poor and rich, can repair to. But is freedom of choice, as a rhetoric, adequate to the hard logic of the population urgencies that face America and the world today? For with dwindling resources and increasing pollution and cluttering technology, the population problem is no longer a matter of option by the individual mother for the individual family. It has become a matter of national, even global, necessity.

The new insight can run in terms of the difference between birth control—which rests on the rights and freedom of the individual—and population control, which rests on the necessities of the nation and therefore on the obligations of the individual. We can no longer assume that population control can operate by letting each person make personal choices, and hoping that they will somehow add up to the national or global good. This was the philosophy behind Adam Smith's "unseen hand of God," as he applied it to the theory of the free market, whereby each individual pursued his own good and thereby assured the common good. Laissez faire was always an appealing idea for human society, provided we could afford the luxury of it. Given the cruel pressures toward sexual conformity in the era of Victorian morals, and the iron trap of the taboos, laissez faire in the birth decisions—free choice to breed or not

to breed, and open access to contraception and abortion—was a necessary and exhilarating phase of the total
struggle for population control as well as for civilized
dignity. It was the liberation phase, and it carried with
it the excitement of all liberation movements.

Liberation rarely leads to restraint, but in this case
it did, and thereby confounded the demographic experts.
A birth turnabout took place in the 1971 figures for the
U.S. that marked a turning point in American population
history. Not only did the birth rate closely approach the
ZPG figure. There were even more important indices.
The marriage age rose. The expectation of family size
dropped: Among younger women in 1955 the expectation was for 3.2 children, in 1967 for 2.9, in 1971 for
2.4—a trend that I venture to call the revolution of
declining expectations. Abortion clinics were opened as
liberal state abortion laws like New York's came into
operation. Male vasectomies increased sharply.

In retrospect, it is easy to explain why this turnabout came about. The devoted efforts of the family
planning movement had much to do with it. But these
efforts were of long standing. They came to fruition,
suddenly and strikingly, at the point where they converged with four other movements. One was the sexual
revolution, which dissociated the hedonic from the reproductive in the sexual act, leading to a new hedonism
that made the old "free love" movement licit and accepted rather than illicit and underground. Part of this
revolution was what I should call the new cognizance

of sexuality, in a hitherto undreamt proliferation of research into sexuality and sexual behavior as well as the anti-natal technology (pill, loop, abortion). The old puritan syndrome—repression plus guilt plus a high birth rate—was turned around into a new formula of hedonism plus acceptance plus a low birth rate. The second was the women's revolution, feeding on the first, but with other sources of strength as well, all leading to a new assertive independence for a woman as a woman (job, career, non-marriage as option, open sexuality, open contraception and abortion, shared options about children and shared care of them). The third was the commune movement, tending toward an extended or joint family, in which the pressure toward the children imperative in every nuclear family was somewhat relieved, and children (at a lesser total birth rate) could be shared, tended, and reared together. The fourth was the ecology movement, which sharpened the logic of population control by adding the specter of a polluted (because crowded) environment and an exhaustion of resources.

These all mark changes in attitudes and values. But it is such changes, rather than laws, censorship, or preachings, which have a powerful impact on birth rates. We learned about this during the New Deal days when despair among the young turned to hope, and led to the postwar period of the "baby boom." We learned about it again in the latter half of the sixties, when family planning converged with hedonic sexuality, the women's revolution, the communes, and the ecological revolution. These were all passionate cultural movements, and their interactive impact was greater and faster than the sum of them taken singly.

Yet, from the standpoint of population control, there are disturbing aspects that need coping with.

The most obvious is the question of dynamics. The change in birth rate and expectation rate was achieved without government say-so, by a change of attitude and belief on the part of the people, about what comes first and what second. This is the ideal way for changes to come about, and it shows that American society is still flexible. But will the same voluntary and spontaneous methods complete the process of virtually stopping population growth?

Because the post-World War II babies have now reached child-bearing age, and will be bearing children for some years, the historically low birth rate must be calculated on a child-bearing population base that is historically high. In this perspective a stabilized (optimal) population will not be achieved until well into the next century, with an addition of perhaps 70 million people by that time. Even if the birth rate during the seventies falls (as it may do) below the 2.11 rate that is the ZPG replacement level, the continued population growth will present problems of crowding, pollution, resources, and social costs. If the rate—due to incalculable changes in public attitudes and life values—wavers in its decline or even starts upward again, the problems will be graver and more urgent.

A second disturbing aspect involves the distribution of population growth. This is not, as some would have it, a qualitative question, but one of continuity of quantitative composition and balance. In every society the poor and less well-educated, those living in urban and rural ghettos and in rural enclaves, tend to have higher fertility rates, while at higher income and educational levels the fertility rate falls. This applies, of course, to every low-income and low-schooling group—black, Puerto Rican, Spanish-American, Appalachian whites, low-income white ethnics.

It is complicated in the U.S. by two other factors. First, for historic rather than genetic reasons, the low-income, low-schooling levels are heavily represented among nonwhites. Second, there is a strong Catholic population, particularly among the white ethnics, which brings in the added factor of the continuing prohibition against birth control and abortion in Catholic doctrine. Thus, the factors of ethnicity and religious belief cut across the various strata of income and education.

It would be highly unrealistic to ignore this thicket of complexities, or to believe that they will disappear by wishing them away. It would also be unrealistic to ignore the intensity of emotion that has been generated here. On the part of the nonwhites there is fear of "genocide" and of white resistance to the growing movements for nonwhite power; on the part of the whites, there is fear of becoming in time a white enclave in a nonwhite population sea. On the part of the Catholics, there is a bruised feeling that the concept of social freedom is hemming in the freedom of Catholics to bear children at their own rate and raise them in their own way, and is doing violence to their cherished doctrines, especially the sanctity of human life; on the part of non-Catholics, there is the fear that Catholics are not only making their own choices, but seeking to thrust them on the rest of the community.

Anyone with some knowledge of how fragile is the cohesiveness of a multi-racial pluralist democratic society will be concerned not only about the hot rhetoric and cold logic of population control, but also about what course is most prudent in the short run and wisest in the long run. Tread lightly and nimbly, we walk on volcanic lava.

At the hearings of the Commission on Population Growth, several of the spokesmen for nonwhites raised the fertility-and-power issue. Reverend Jesse Jackson: "Virtually all the security we have is in the number of children we produce." Naomi Gray: "If this ecology movement talks about fewer people, the question of who gets to survive is raised." And Manuel Aragon, appearing for the Spanish-speaking people: "What we must do is to encourage large Mexican-American families so that we will eventually be so numerous that the system will either respond or be overwhelmed."

Something of the same fear of nonwhite genocide, and assertion of the will to fertility, will be found throughout the developing world. One thinks of the 1968 episode when Robert McNamara, as head of the World Bank, had to be rescued by helicopter from an angry crowd at the Calcutta airport. The whole world ecology movement, including not only population control but environmental reform and the setting of limits to economic growth, is seen as part of a more or less conscious continuance of the colonial mentality. Thus, William Banage, heading the Ugandan delegation to the Stockholm conference: "Our fundamental environment problem is how to raise the material standard of life of our people to levels that are humanly decent."

One answer is, of course, that no people—developing or developed—can raise its living standard so long as it is caught in the tragic trap between mouths to feed and whatever there is to feed them with. The premise of the population movement is that hostility to fertility control is allayed as living standards and educational levels rise.

This is suggested by several studies about black attitudes and behavior. A Commission poll found that among the blacks themselves over 85 percent see population growth as a problem for the whole nation, and 35 percent see it as a serious problem. Another study, for the Planned Parenthood group, shows that between 1966 and 1970 the fertility rate among black women in the poverty category dropped 26 percent, from 186 to 137 births per thousand. But there are other, less heartening figures. In the general population of women dropouts below the high-school level the birthrate was 3.9, of which almost a third were unwanted children. But among similar black women dropouts it was 5.2, with more than half unwanted.

There is a lack of sensitivity among whites about the sources of black enragement. If they studied the nonwhite death rates, which have improved considerably but are still bleak, they might understand somewhat better why the blacks are not overeager to stifle a compensatory fertility rate. Irrational? Yes, especially if we remember that the high fertility rate adds to the wretchedness of their living conditions, which in turn re-enforces their death rate. But this is an area riddled with irrationals. Meanwhile those who rest their hope and dream on voluntary controls point to the fact that with each additional year of completed school experience and work experience, black earnings increase beyond the increase among whites. If this sort of differential gain leads to a continued rise in educational and living standard levels, and therefore to less bitterness about population controls, the voluntary way may prove best. But if the black bitterness continues and the differential fertility rate is sustained, it will lead to an enragement of the other Americans who have responded to the appeals to practice fertility restraint. In that case, as in the similar event of continued enragement between Catholics and non-Catholics, the dream of the family planners will shiver into dust.

For that dream was a good weapon for fighting

puritan repressions, but it isn't a good one for getting total acceptance of voluntary restraints, nor for fighting the group tensions that stand in the way of achieving a stabilized population level, without so badly skewed a distribution as to feed the socially divisive resentments and rages.

In the phase now ending, there have been several major clusters of resistance to fertilty control. I give them roughly in an ascending order of importance. First, the Great Power illusion, that higher birth rates are the sinews of war strength. Those who pursued pro-natalist national policies on this assumption were building on a myth. Second, the resistance from the rural life style in many parts of the world where peasants want more children (especially male) for help on the soil, and where the woman is fearful of her social image as an undutiful or undesired sexual partner if she should seem deficient in giving her mate a huddle of children.

Third, the religious resistances, notably (as I have already mentioned) from Catholics but not always. While the Church hierarchy still clings to pro-natalist doctrines, it has been undermined by a rebellion of the lower clergy, and in practice by a quiet but determined refusal of many church members to go along with the ban on contraception. Fourth, there are the political-ethnic resistances, especially from Marxist and Third World nations, and from elites of color in Africa and Asia who scorn to ride along with a white-inspired Western movement. I have already discussed the impact of this strain of thinking on attitudes inside the U.S. Yet, the current campaign of fertility control in China is only the latest instance of the triumph of practical policies over the chimeras of theory and the nightmarish suspicions born of centuries of oppression and hate. From Russia to China, from India to Jamaica, the practical rulers strive earnestly (if not always mightily) to set some limits to the galloping destructiveness of the birth rate.

I add, fifthly, an overall resistance factor that (at least in the West) has been historically more crucial than any of the above, but has now been all but overcome. I mean, of course, the hypocritical ethos and value system of the dominant ruling classes—not the ignorant, wretched, and benighted, but the affluent, the respectable, the "educated" and "enlightened" solid citizens. I am speaking of the seamier and more repressive side of what we call the "Protestant ethos" (which was Catholic and Jewish as well), of the "virtuous codes" of eighteenth and early nineteenth century Britain and America, of the "respectable morality" of the Victorian era in both countries.

If ever we had reason to invoke a pox on a dominant value system, for the shadow it cast over the lives of ordinary men and women, it is this one. It saw the sexual act as covert and dirty, linked it only with the propagation of children, regarded any effort to dissociate the two as immoral and vicious. It tried to strip the hedonic from the relations of men and women and thus doomed them either to an intolerable burden of child-rearing, often under wretched conditions, or to a loveless life in which sexual pleasure was suspect and warmth of human contact was congealed. I have spoken before of the cluster of sexual revolutions that have made this ethos largely archaic, despite its blue-nosed survivals. But a young generation that has freed itself from these dominant codes finds it hard to recapture the spell they exerted over centuries of "civilized" living.

We also tend to forget that the road of release from this repressive puritanism took two forks. One was toward anti-natal attitudes based on the new sense of freedom, the other on an earthy celebration of life, based on the same sense of freedom, but child-centered rather than childless-centered.

At this point, a personal word that may illustrate some of the problems population control must still face. I write this with at least a dash of contriteness, although I don't beat my breast abjectly and have no pathogenic scars of conscience about it. I have myself been married twice, and have had three children by each marriage. Thus, I am one of the philoprogenitive tribe, with the image of the Old Testament patriarch as my self-image. I like the feel of children, their clatter and clutter, and as mine have grown up and left on life-courses of their own, with only one still marginally present in our home, I miss them. They in turn have been strangely and affectionately tolerant of my foibles.

I now believe, in my upper cortical centers, that

six children are too many and a violation of Kant's cate-
gorical imperative, as well as of all the precepts from the
early Malthusian fathers to the latest proponents of zero
population growth. But I mention my propagative past
to suggest that my more rational present view comes
from no personality need of my own, no death-against-
life glacial bleakness of emotion such as one sometimes
finds, alas, in the more febrile anti-natal crusaders. It
comes rather from the considered facts about the human
race and its urgencies and prospects.

These facts and prospects have been mooted for
some years, and have become common knowledge during the last five. They are the crowding of people on our
continent and planet, the cult and dominance of technology, the pollutions that have resulted, and long riffling
of the environment, the congestion of living, the decline
in the quality of life, the drain of resources, the throttling
of the highways, the defacing of the landscape, the
strain on medical and educational facilities, the frightening chances of world famine.

I must go back here to pick up an earlier thread of
analysis—the fault-line between the rhetoric and logic
of any social movement. The rhetoric of this one still
operates on the freedom-and-persuasion principle, and
hopes that the campaign of history from now on will be
similar to what it has been, and that past victories
presage future ones. The logic of the facts themselves
points to the need for a change in the underlying concept, from the assumption of freedom to the use of the

collective will, and for the possibility that carrot-and-stick tactics may be necessary, including bonuses and other inducements, and both social and legal pressures.

From the assumption that freedom of choice will solve everything, we shall have to make a Copernican change to the assumption that the right to breed can no longer be seen as an absolute right but can be exercised only within the frame of felt needs in the society and the world. The right to breed, practiced for so many centuries without limits, must now be pursued within limits. For when man is himself close to being an endangered species, absolute rights are an intolerable luxury. Ideally these limits should be drawn voluntarily, by the individual. But a society has the right to limit the extent to which a person—deliberately or thoughtlessly, for pleasure, prestige, pride, patriotism, ethnic commitment, absent-mindedness, or the hope of immortality—can bring children into the world as a burden on its resources, its social systems, its ecological systems, its living space, and the quality of its life.

If we recognize this, we can define the third phase of population control into which we are now moving. It is like nothing dreamt of by the neo-Malthusian reformers. It bursts the bounds of the universe of the present family planners. For it brings in the ugly specter of social and governmental coercion. It raises the question of whether there can be collective American action—and beyond that, collective world action—to limit the growth of population and its related factors and keep them in balance. To put it differently, can there be—in this stormy area—a collective American will? Even harder, can there be a collective world will? Or, must the reliance continue to be, as in the second phase, on freedom, individual conscience, and education?

I put this in the form of questions, because we are not anywhere near finding the answers. But a new phase in the history of any movement is begun when new questions are formulated. We have taken an important step when we discover that the answers we had for old questions are no longer valid—not that they are the wrong answers, but that they are now the wrong questions.

Take my own case, as an Old Testament patriarch. I was operating on the old rhetoric of freedom of parental choice. I felt confident not only that we wanted our children, but that we would be able to rear them, educate them, watch over them, and give them a start in life. Then the social climate changed. The new element that was invoked was conscience: Even though parents want children, and can rear them tolerably well, can they in good conscience add intolerably to the burdens of the society? If I were doing it all again, I should probably accept the mandate of conscience, and say, No.

But how many will accept this mandate of conscience? Not only how many individuals, but how many ethnic and religious groups inside our community? And how many nations in the world community? I have spoken of the problems of conscience faced by Catholic mothers and fathers, as well as the decisions of the hierarchy. I have also spoken of the prides, hurts, and enragements of nonwhites in America. One could add that with the spread of affluence—and assuming a continuing strong parental drive—there will be many more families able to give their children good rearing, and while they will not have sprawling families, they may balk at voluntarily restricting themselves to only two.

In the world community there is bound to be, as I have suggested, considerable skepticism about following a West-oriented mandate of conscience. Thus, at the Stockholm world conference on the environment, the Chinese delegation explained that the pollution from China's nuclear testing was defensive, a socialist pollution, as compared with the "blackmailing fall-out arising from super-power hegemony." And if the Algerian delegation speaks for other Third World nations in saying that the environmental problem arises from "capitalism, imperialism, and racialism," the chances of reaching a world consensus on population control seem dubious enough.

This is precisely the lion in the path of all dreams of population control, by those who have some optimal balance of population in mind, some "stationary state," and who fondly believe it can be accomplished by education and freedom. The lion in the path is the indifference of those who have not been won over, by education or conscience, and the active hostility of those who feel that the dream is not dreamt for them—that actually it is being dreamt against them—and who will not therefore fit themselves snugly into the plans of the population planners.

✦ For myself, in my own value scheme, I detest government coercions in the areas of life-choices that ought to remain private. If I can indulge a hope, it is that we should achieve a minor and manageable rate of population growth by social pressures, rather than governmental action. But I don't fool myself into confusing hope and reality. It is true that the climate of opinion has changed drastically. Where once the opinion pressures and social pressures were toward having children if you wanted sex, today they are the other way—toward having sex without children, or rather toward having maximal sex and minimal progeny. But it is also true that this climate applies now only to a spreading minority—at best, to a narrow majority; and that you can't generate real social pressures to carry through a population control program unless those pressures come from the overwhelming majority—and unless they have been internalized, as the anti-sexual and pro-natal taboos were once internalized.

✦ The case history of Japan is very much in point. At first sight it seems to offer proof that a nation can cut its fertility rate sharply and stabilize its population by drastic governmental controls. But a closer look shows that the Japanese achieved it less through political coercion than through the basic structure of their society. Japanese society is a closely knit set of highly cohesive social clusters—the family, the corporation, the trade union, the political faction, the political party, the university, the Army, the skill groups, the nation. Once the directives had been decided upon, at the higher power levels, the problem of translating them into action through general acceptance was a problem only of supplying adequate incentives and touching the springs of social habit among a people accustomed both to directed stability and directed drastic change. The basic method was the organized availability of anti-fertility technology and clinics, and the widespread campaign for abortions and sterilization. Every agency of Japanese life worked in a coordinated way to achieve it, according to a carefully formulated plan.

Japan's relatively homogeneous population was an important factor: A multi-racial and highly pluralist society would lack this advantage. Japan's traditionalism and cohesion, and its cluster of loyalty systems, were more important. There are no case histories to suggest that a society as different from the Japanese as America's would be equally effective in the same campaign. Unlike America, Japan's problem now is that its drive to cut population may have been too successful, in the sense that there is a serious shortage of skilled labor, a declining number of young people entering the labor market, and a strong upward thrust of wages that may impair Japan's competitive advantage in the world market.

A society like the American would have to use other means. For those beyond the reach of majority social pressures, there would have to be the "carrot" incentives. Some have suggested non-baby bonuses, others have talked of bounties for vasectomies, still others have proposed marketable licenses for babies that could be sold by the poor to the rich, thereby achieving not only a more stable population but also a redistribution of wealth; the poor would grow richer by having to raise fewer children, and the rich would get poorer by having to raise so many. While I have no objection in principle to the carrot technique, I fear it would run up against huge psychological obstacles. The campaign for vasectomies would succeed mainly with the converted, not with those who would quickly call it a white genocidal plot against nonwhites. The same applies to marketable baby licenses, which would mostly embitter the low-income groups who already feel that life's chances are distributed according to gradations of wealth.

The use of the draft during the Civil War, when the poor sold themselves as draft proxies to the rich, led to serious riots and left a scar on the national conscience. I suspect this might prove true of these devices I describe, so long as they go counter to deeply held convictions in the society.

There may be a different way out of the dilemmas of population control. Part of the new third phase is the shifting of emphasis from population itself to the total global environment, of which population is only one factor. The Club of Rome's approach to the whole problem, through systems analysis, has come to be widely

debated, as has a recent British report along the same
lines. At M.I.T. Jay Forester has developed what he
calls "System Dynamics," by which he feeds data on
the crucial factors of a changing total system into com-
puters and projects their interactions.

In the case of the world environment, what has
emerged is a pentagon of major factors, with population
one of the five. The others are technology and industrial
growth, food consumption, natural and energy resources,
and pollution rate. The projections made by the Club of
Rome study—in a book called *The Limits to Growth,* by
D. H. Meadows and an M.I.T. team—conjure up a
gloomy, end-of-the-world picture by the year 2,000.

One doesn't have to accept these particular projections, which have been severely criticized for the data
themselves, in order to find value in the total systems
approach. It offers a new perspective on population control. Already one of the leading American environ-
mentalists, Barry Commoner, has attacked the ZPG
champion, Paul Ehrlich, for overemphasizing population
at the expense of the role of technology, which Commoner regards as the principal polluter. There will be
other similar feuds in the period of intellectual history
ahead, as we debate which aspect of the multiple problem needs to be attacked with the greatest intensity. But
what is important is the new emerging logic—that population is linked not only with food supply but with
technology, energy resources, pesticides, pollution rates,
and economic growth itself, in a fateful live-or-die com-

bination. If you also see it linked, as I suggested earlier, with the sexual revolution, the women's revolution, the commune movement, and the changes in the value system, you begin to get a sense of the sheer complexity of what lies ahead—but also a sense of what you can draw upon, in moving toward a manageable balance.

I stress both the adjective and noun in the last phrase I have used. It is a balance we are striving for—a balance between all the major factors, a new balance for the world that will be the global equivalent of an individual's homeostasis. And it is not some absolute we are striving for, nor an "optimal" population level we have dreamt up, or have arrived at by a computer: It is something merely manageable, something we can grapple with and live with, in an imperfect world.

It is for this reason that I don't go along with the "end of growth" school in the economic realm any more than I go along with those who want the total end of population growth. In social organisms, to end growth means to risk stagnation. It is growth at an exponential rate that is the enemy, and which can become a metastasis. Slow, rational, controlled, and balanced growth is not only manageable, but it also provides the vitality that every organism needs. For where there is runaway growth, every problem becomes a runaway problem—as we are now witnessing; where there is no growth, every problem becomes a sticky problem; where there is controlled growth, every problem becomes a manageable problem.

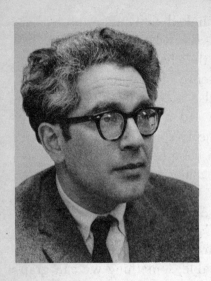

Dr. Nathan Glazer has been an authority in such problem areas as urban social policy and ethnic and race relations for more than twenty years. After a long tenure as Professor of Sociology at the University of California, Berkeley, Dr. Glazer accepted the post of Professor of Education and Social Structure at Harvard University. His entry into the world of academia was preceded by an eventful year as Urban Sociologist for the U. S. Government's Housing and Home Finance Agency.

In 1963, Dr. Glazer was co-author with Daniel P. Moynihan of BEYOND THE MELTING POT, which won the Anisfield-Wolf Award. He has written a number of other important works, including THE LONELY CROWD and STUDIES IN HOUSING AND MINORITY GROUPS. He writes regularly for the NEW YORK TIMES SUNDAY MAGAZINE, COMMENTARY MAGAZINE, and THE PUBLIC INTEREST.

Nathan Glazer

IT SO HAPPENS that this article is being written in Nagpur, in Maharashtra State, India. Nagpur is a city of almost one million, formerly a state capital of the Central Provinces, as they were then called. They are now Madhya Pradesh, and Nagpur is now a provincial city, oversupplied with the buildings needed for a state capital in India. Nagpur, just as many other Indian cities, has grown rapidly. Like many other Indian cities, it is a rather less pleasant place to live for the well-to-do, and probably even the poor, than it was twenty years ago. The sidewalks and streets are inevitably more neglected than formerly—crumbling in the older parts, not yet built in the newer parts. The schools and colleges are overcrowded. Many of the students are from the Scheduled Castes, who are now favored for admission by national and state policy by reserved seats and stipends. Where large bungalows once stood in enormous and well-kept grounds, one finds the bungalow itself badly maintained, the grounds shabby and encroached upon by shacks, squatters, and new buildings. The rivers are places for the disposal of garbage and where squatters resort for their water needs.

One could continue the description. And one could conclude that the problems of Nagpur are owing to population growth, which, even though less in India than in some developing countries, has been sufficient to increase the population no less than 25 percent in ten years—adding something like 108 million people to the population of India, with every prospect that that number will be even higher in the next ten years.

Certainly India is the best case one could imagine for population control, most public leaders agree. A substantial if only doubtfully effective program of family planning receives government support, and almost every educated Indian seems to place population growth in the first place among the many problems facing India.

And yet, even in India, looking at the specific problems of Nagpur, one can make a case that population growth, while undoubtedly a very severe problem, is not to be blamed for all the problems of Nagpur. Consider, for example, the overcrowded colleges into which Indian students are desperately trying to gain admission this year, and their declining quality, which was expressed in Nagpur last year by a campaign of mass copying in the university exams. The fact is, the overcrowding is owing less to an increase in birth rate as such than to the fact that much greater numbers of persons, in statuses that previously never dreamed of going to college, now want to go, and many of them receive some modest government support for going. Population growth has something to do with the overcrowding and the declining standards. But the push to equality, which expresses itself in India through special programs for Scheduled Castes and tribes, certainly has as much to do with it.

Another factor that is responsible for the huge increase in the number of colleges and their declining quality is the fact that college seems to be the only way to get a good job. Consider the case of the medical schools, which have grown rapidly, but far from enough to accommodate all the students who wish to go. Indian doctors are not paid well, but they are somewhat better paid than others. Medical education also offers the opportunity for emigration to the United Kingdom, Canada, the United States, and other countries in which there is a high demand for doctors and high pay for them. Considering these factors and others, can one say that the crowding in the Indian medical schools is owing to population growth? Not exactly—it is owing, if one looks at proximate causes, to a stagnant economy that offers few opportunities, and that thus leads many to take the path to a somewhat better income and the chance for emigration.

The squatter colonies are the best demonstration, one would think, that India's problems are owing to overpopulation. No one could argue with this. But once again, the proximate cause seems to be poverty and governmental inefficiency. There is plenty of space in and around Nagpur. It is not expensive, in world terms, to provide what is considered decent housing for poor Indians. It is rather more expensive, it is true, to provide water and sanitary facilities. What seems lacking in their provision? Certainly not manpower—there is vast unemployment. Capital goods, certainly. Organization, definitely. What India suggests is not that population growth is not a problem, for it most definitely is. At the crudest level, one can see what a problem it is when one discovers that the cook, who earns perhaps two hundred rupees a month, has ten children and seems young enough to have more. Inevitably, each is doomed to a degree of poverty and a limitation of opportunities far greater than one or two children would face. Nationally, one sees it when one sees the enormous figures on the requirements for classrooms and teachers that are necessary in a country where 14 million potential new scholars are added to the population each year—as against a fifth of that in the prosperous United States.

But one must add other things to explain the overcrowding in institutions and the prevailing air of neglect and shabbiness in Nagpur. One must add, first of all, an overwhelming poverty, which is itself not exclusively the product of population growth. One must add the drive toward equality. One must add the set of values that lead the best educated to avoid the difficult course of work in the villages and the countryside, and to take instead the course that may lead to the civil service or to emigration. One must add the quality of government, which, even in India, leads some cities, with similar resources, to be rather better managed and maintained than others.

But is not the population problem the one problem most amenable to change through governmental intervention and action? One wonders whether it is not as refractory as all the others—and in the end dependent on change in the others in large measure if it is to be effective. Thus, a more efficient governmental machinery would clearly assist family planning in being effective. More trained people willing to work in the villages and the slums of the cities would be necessary, and less who eagerly seek the safe haven of an easy government job or emigration. A reduction in poverty would paradoxically be required in order to reduce the population growth that contributes so substantially to it—for the reduction in poverty would open to more people the thought that their lives *could* be different, and the further thought that their lives could be improved if they reduced the number of their children. Universal education for the school-aged, from which India is still far, would reduce population, because it would make education for family planning more effective, and because it would teach parents that they could no longer depend on the tiny contribution that even small children working can bring to family income in India.

Even this sketchy discussion is enough to suggest the way population growth forms a complex together with poverty, values, government, and that an exclusive concentration on population growth as a means to overcoming poverty is not likely to be effective. India, where there has been a concentration on curbing population growth, shows no marked success in moving out of abysmal poverty, or in achieving a lower rate of population growth. Other nations, such as Brazil and Mexico, where there have been no government programs of population control, have shown greater success in at least becoming more prosperous. What this suggests is not that Brazil and Mexico do not need population control programs nor that India should abandon its program, but rather that other changes seem to be required to begin the move out of abysmal poverty, and these other changes may themselves be essential to the success of family control programs.

India provides other food for thought in considering population problems and population control. It is remarkable how inappropriate are some of the suggestions raised in presumably the best-informed quarters in an attempt to control population growth. For example: It is proposed that the age of marriage be raised to eighteen, or even twenty-one. (The average age of marriage is now sixteen.) It is, however, never suggested how this is to be enforced. Or, what girls in the villages of India are expected to do between puberty and eighteen or twenty-one. The fact is the age of marriage is hardly controlled by law—though at the margin there may well be some influence. It is controlled by social considerations. In a society in which there are jobs for young women, they may marry later. In a society where they are expected to go to school until the age of eighteen or twenty, another factor is introduced that delays the age of marriage. In a society in which new values develop in which young women want to be free to experience new things such as travel without the burden of children, again the age of marriage is higher. One may think of other factors. None of these prevail in the villages of India, where there are neither jobs for women, education for women beyond a minimal few elementary years—and this only if one is lucky—and certainly no new values that would lead to such ideas as travel for pleasure. These do exist to a modest extent in the cities, and particularly for the upper middle classes—and there indeed, one does see an increase in the age of marriage for girls.

The major thrust of the Indian family planning program has been the provision of loops and other contraceptives to women, and of condoms and vasectomies to men, through the agency of medical and paramedical personnel. One again asks, Is this likely to be effective when the *only* contact of villagers with medical and paramedical personnel may be in connection with family planning? When resort to doctors and drugs and the like is part of one's life, then contraception provided by doctors may become part of one's life, too. When it is not, it is hardly likely that this one area of medical practice can flourish in the absence of every other. One will not have the habits that lead to recourse to the doctor or nurse, or the habits that lead to the regular taking of some drug or medicine, or the trust in the medical personnel that is necessary to take their admonitions seriously. Once again, one sees the interrelatedness of a number of key elements—and the near futility or inefficiency of concentration on one feature in the control of population.

India offers one other example of a phenomenon of importance in population control. The results of the Indian census of 1971 as to gross population growth, broken down by religion, have recently been published. It turned out that in 1961-71, the Muslims grew more rapidly than the Hindus, though the Christians and Sikhs grew more rapidly than either. Immediately there were expressions of alarm by Hindu spokesmen and letters-to-the-editor writers: By simple extrapolation the population of India, now some 10 percent Muslim, would become majority Muslim in four hundred years or so!

It is unnecessary to point out the naiveté of such calculations. No social phenomenon remains constant for anything like four hundred years. Obviously something will happen long before that. Indeed, if the rates of population growth of Hindus and Muslims remain constant for another hundred years, it is possible most Indians will be dead of starvation or plague and the issue of the triumph numerically of Muslims in the following three hundred years will become purely academic.

Is all this relevant to the problems of the advanced nations? In these countries population growth rates are half or less that of India, but each additional person requires a complement of investment for physical infrastructure and social and health and educational services and consumption that would possibly serve one hundred Indians. Further, in these countries literacy is universal, and the entire population can be reached by the most advanced communications media in the world.

Oddly enough, a good deal of Indian experience *is* relevant to advanced nations.

First of all, many of the problems we ascribe to population growth in the United States are the effect of the movement to equality. When we hear complaints that Yosemite is overcrowded, that the recreation facilities in the wilderness no longer provide peace and quiet, we shouldn't conclude that it is because the population is rapidly increasing. That is only part of the story. It is also because the population is becoming more prosperous and demanding the facilities that were once reserved for the wealthy. In India, in contrast, one may see that certain luxurious facilities have no problem of overcrowding at all, because all too few can afford them. It is similar with the rapid growth of colleges and universities and the complaints of how hard it is to get into exclusive colleges as against thirty years ago. Certainly population growth has played a part. But a much larger part has been played by the growth in equality, which means that 50 percent of young people of college age now enter college as against 10 percent a few decades back; and that egalitarian principles affect elite institutions, which are now open to all, as against only the children of the elite. Many of the complaints against crowding are thus only complaints against the fact that more and more people can enjoy what only a few enjoyed. Admittedly, as more enjoy these facilities, all enjoy them less. There seems no simple answer to this problem. One cannot easily multiply a few more Cape Cods or Yosemites or Harvards. One simply must come to terms with the revolution for equality, which still has the capacity to transform many more elite institutions than it has yet touched.

Yet another group of unpleasant social features we ascribe to population growth can, as in India, be ascribed to poverty. First of all, population growth itself, even in the richer countries, is still associated with poverty, even though their poverty is radically different from that of India. (If the average American disposes of one hundred times the resources available to the average Indian, the average poor American probably disposes of one thousand times the resources available to the average poor Indian, for the average poor American, after all, has access to the pure water of a very expensive water supply system, the flush toilets of a very expensive sanitary system, the schools of a very expensive educational system, the doctors and hospitals of a very expensive health-care system, housing that is generally equivalent to that which only wealthy Indians have access to, etc.) Poverty even in the richest countries still seems associated with an incapacity to look ahead to foresee the depressing effect of many children on family life and welfare, and control one's behavior thereby. We no longer have in rich countries the incentive to family growth of the pitiful earnings of working children, but we do have the incentive of the fact that each child means more benefits on welfare. Thus, poverty itself is a problem in rich countries. It contributes to unaesthetic aspects of environment—garbage in the streets, crowding in the houses, inadequate maintenance—and to other features that many ascribe too crudely to "population explosion," as well as, through some features of poverty itself, to the multiplication of pointlessly large families directly.

Finally, one further feature of the Indian situation finds a parallel in the American: the involvement of population control with the conflict of races and ethnic groups. Thus, black militants attack family planning facilities in the ghettoes as "genocide." One notes that a number of Jewish writers have pointed with concern to the very low birth rate of the Jewish population (if it were higher than the average American birth rate, rather than the reverse, one can be sure some non-Jews would be alarmed). I doubt that these political considerations really affect population growth. It seems hardly likely that black women will allow militants to limit their freedom to limit their children, or that Jewish families will start having larger families in response to the evidence that the American Jewish population is not reproducing itself. Yet, under certain circumstances these political factors can have an influence. If militants are strong enough to frighten away family planning agencies from locating in black areas, that will limit the ability of black women to receive information, drugs, and devices. The statistics show that black population growth is less than that of Mexican Americans and Puerto Ricans. The latter is undoubtedly a source of satisfaction to the more simple-minded militants in those groups, and they will undoubtedly do what they can to keep this state of affairs constant—though once again, social causation is so complex that we can expect them to fail.

But the experience of India and other developing nations is only of limited relevance to the United States and the rest of the developed world. In a word, the difference is that in the United States most of the population is capable of being influenced by information, and capable of taking relevant action under the influence of that information. This, alas, is far from the case in India. In the United States, family decisions to have children are in large measure rational, in some sense—they respond to such calculations as the state of the economy, the income of the family, the wife's desire to work, the desires of the husband and wife to live in a certain style. There are influences that in some sense are "nonrational" but in other senses are quite rational: for example, the influence of the large families of the Kennedys, which undoubtedly contributed to the fashion of large families among the educated and affluent in the sixties. I call such a decision "rational" in that it is not purely a reflection of traditional patterns that dictate accepting God's gift of children, regardless of numbers and impact. It is based on such considerations as wanting to be fashionable, or believing large families to have a desirable style of life. The fashion itself is only possible because of the mass media and their saturation coverage of events, which reached and influenced vast numbers with the story of the Kennedys. Finally, another rational aspect is that the fashion, when it influences persons, can be implemented by the proper means, such as stopping birth-control measures.

It is because of such rational influences on people's behavior in the United States that one sees such large swings in the birth rate, as against the painfully slow decline in India. The birth rate is no longer a "natural" phenomenon, a phenomenon in "nature," in the United States. It is in large measure owing to the rational decisions of millions of people reflecting large social influences. In India, perhaps a few percent of births reflect such rational decisions; in the United States, on the contrary, perhaps half or more births reflect rational decisions to have children. Ideally, we would want 100 percent of births to reflect such decisions.

Under such circumstances—and we can come close to achieving them by such measures as a free distribution of birth-control information, universal education in birth control, and abortion on demand—would we have reason to be concerned with the problem of population growth in advanced nations? I believe under circumstances in which nearly 100 percent of births were owing to rational decisions, population growth could be controlled without the measures of compulsion that science-fiction writers propose and so many of us fear may be necessary—licenses for the right to have children, a market in such licenses, state-sponsored infanticide for transgressors, etc. For I believe population growth under conditions of universal literacy, mass communication, and free choice would be responsive to the news of population growth itself. Thus, in recent years we have seen a surprising drop in the rate of population growth in the United States. Undoubtedly this is owing to many influences. In the first place, one would have to put economic recession. But undoubtedly other influences have played a role: easier abortion, more accessible birth-control information and devices, the cultural changes that have led to the rise in the age of marriage of men and women, more women working, the rise in the price of single family homes, women's lib, and so on. But among these influences, in no matter how modest a position, I would place the view that population growth should not proceed unchecked, and that zero population growth is a necessary and desirable goal. This general point of view is now commonly accepted. It is no longer radical, exotic, or unfashionable. One recalls that Robert Kennedy, committed to family planning, used to apologize for the size of his family, one indication of the change between the earlier and the later sixties. We are now accustomed to very rapid changes in public opinion; something that is seen as a serious problem by very few people suddenly comes to be accepted as a serious problem by very many people, indeed enough to create new social movements, new habits, and new legislation. This has happened in the sixties with ecology, with women's liberation, and with population growth. The preconditions for such rapid and influential changes in public opinion are mass literacy, effective mass communication, the openness of people to new information, and their willingness to change on the basis of new information.

I am not arguing that the present drop in the rate of American population growth is owing solely to the movement to arouse people to the dangers of population growth, or that we will not see again a rise in the rate of population growth. However, even if we do see another rise, the long-range trend must be for the awareness of the dangers of population growth to become ever more widespread and influential, and for this awareness to become ever more potent as one of the influences affecting population growth. How will this influence work? Not directly. Economists have been all too convincing in demonstrating to us the difference between behavior that benefits oneself directly and behavior that may benefit the world, but in too insignificant a measure if indulged in by the single individual to affect his own action. But this new awareness of the danger of population growth will work through legislation. It has already had an influence in making distribution of contraceptive knowledge widespread in welfare programs. It has had an influence in affecting new legislation easing abortion. This awareness leads us to examine proposed new social legislation from the point of view of its possible incentive to population growth—even though there are dilemmas here we cannot solve easily.

A few years ago Kingsley and Judith Blake Davis argued that even in conditions of free access to contraception and abortion and wide publicity for them the population would grow at more than a zero rate because married couples on the whole preferred three or four children. I believe this preference can itself change, indeed is changing, under the weight of the simple but overwhelming observation that the world cannot afford more than a stable population over the long run. The act of having a large family will more and more be seen as an antisocial act. There will be less and less incentive in tax and social legislation to have large families. The methods to control the size of one's family will become ever easier, accessible, and acceptable.

Admittedly this is an optimistic perspective. It assumes man is rational, if we give him the information and facilities and institutions that encourage rationality.

If I am wrong, we will in the end have to resort to the devices of the science-fiction writers.

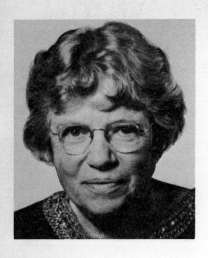

Dr. Margaret Mead's lifelong study of the family of man and her work toward the betterment of the human condition need no introduction. Her contributions in the areas of cultural change and ecology as they relate to family life and mental health have been acknowledged by more awards and honors than can be recounted here, among them the Merrill-Palmer Institute of Human Development and Family Life Citation and the National Achievement Award.

As early as 1949, Associated Press selected her as the Outstanding Woman of the Year in the Field of Science. In 1965, she was chosen as the Outstanding Woman of the Twentieth Century by Nationwide Women Editors. Her many services include curator of ethnology of the Museum of Natural History, Fellow and Chairman of the Committee on Science in the Promotion of Human Welfare, and co-chairman of the U.S. Task Force on the Future of Mankind.

Margaret Mead

THERE IS URGENT NEED for halting the growth of world population, for conservative estimates place world population at approximately 7 billion by the year 2,000. The present population is already putting a heavy strain on the natural environment—destroying beaches and estuaries, killing lakes and rivers, polluting the oceans, and loading the atmosphere with unmanageable debris. Our whole natural environment—the resources on which we depend for life itself, and the specific protections of the climate and habitability of the earth—are endangered.

Population is not, it is true, the only factor that is stressing the environment. The other principal factor is a break in the natural chain: Materials borrowed from the environment for nourishment, clothing, and other manufactured goods are no longer returned again in usable form. New methods of synthesis and of manufacture have broken this chain and stressed the environment with materials that are either unassimilable or actually harmful—threatening to destroy the cloud cover that protects the earth from the fierceness of the sun, raise the temperature of the oceans so that they can no longer cool the earth, produce deterioration in the sources of food supply.

While we may expect that an awareness of these conditions will promote the development of new technologies to remedy some of the present damage and prevent further stressful pollution, the contribution that increased population makes to increased pollution is inescapable. The well-being of this small planet, man's only home, is dependent upon maintaining a balance between population and the natural environment.

Although it can be demonstrated that the increase in population between now and the year 2,000 will place heavy stress on every type of resource, there will still be differences of opinion about the need to reduce the population of particular areas of the earth, of specific countries, and particular parts of countries. Many countries possess vast unoccupied areas. A glance at the map shows population distributed very unequally over the earth's surface, and there are great differences in the density of populations in different parts of the world. For example, the difference between Greenland, which has a population density of 0, and Mongolia, which has a density of 1 per square kilometer; the U.S., which has a density of 57.4 per square mile and Hong Kong and Singapore with densities of 3,955 and 3,528 respectively. Arguments may be advanced for the extreme need to reduce population in certain manifestly overcrowded areas and countries—the newly created independent state of Bangladesh, for example, where the capacity of the area to support its population has already been passed; or for more population in a small, fertile, and relatively unpopulated country like New Zealand.

If world population is to be reduced, however,

every nation must share in the task. It is unfeasible, in the present climate of world opinion, with such tremendous discrepancies between the standard of living of the industrialized, industrializing, and unindustrialized nations, to demand population control from the poorer countries without demanding it from the richer countries. Furthermore, there are urgent reasons for population control at all points on the continuum: in the very poorest countries so that the people may meet minimum requirements for nutrition and shelter, education and medical care—which they are far from doing now; in the moderately affluent countries, so that they may retain their present well-being; and in the very affluent, like the United States, because our high standard of living places an enormous stress on the natural resources of the planet. We are 6 percent of the world population and are estimated to be using up 50 percent of the earth's irreplaceable natural resources. It is also estimated that each child born and reared in the U.S. produces one hundred times the pollution of a child born in India by our use of cars, power, synthetic materials, etc.

The pattern of settlement is itself misleading. As one looks at the map, it looks as if there were ample room for populations to spread beyond their present concentrations. But a long-term study of urbanization reveals a trend toward these great conurbations—such as those in North America on the East and West Coasts, around the Great Lakes, and around the Gulf. These patterns are paralleled in Europe and other parts of the world. The kind of urbanization within which we live and will live in the foreseeable future tends toward such concentrations, so that urban services such as transportation, electric power, delivery of food, etc., can be facilitated. We may be able to change the style of urban life —develop a large number of small communities of diverse types of composition and relative local autonomy— if we provide major services on a continental scale, and include much more green space and even small wildernesses within urban areas. But we have at present small grounds for hope that these great urban areas will not continue to grow at the expense of the more distant countrysides. The need for population control must therefore be seen in terms of the kind of urban patterns, and the attendant dangers of concentrations of smog, water pollution from the wastes of cities; and the social dangers of crowding, noise, and crime that characterize vast, easily traversed areas of settlement.

Furthermore, competition among nation states for population leads to attitudes that promote warfare and strife, and warfare is becoming increasingly insupportable under conditions of modern military destructiveness. Competition for population leads to fear on the part of these less populated or more slowly growing countries, and expansionist policies on the part of the more crowded and rapidly growing countries. On the other hand, competition between countries over the extent to which they can bring their populations in balance with their resources can lead to the kind of mutual rivalry and comparison of relative well-being and prosperity that promotes the well-being of each population, and discourages an interest in destructive competition and war.

Gross comparisons of population lead almost inevitably to feelings of inferiority on the part of smaller countries unless they are compensated for, as in Scandinavia, for example, by a very high level of well-being for the entire population. If the countries of the world are compared on the basis of the ratio among the relevant factors of land and other resources, population and the health, education, and welfare of the people, the smaller countries, within different technological levels, come off very well. Among the industrialized countries, however, the well-being of a considerable proportion of the population in the United States comes off very poorly. The U.S. is tenth in infant death rate, for example, and has several million people at almost starvation level, a large amount of illiteracy, and tremendous malnutrition and misery.

A further factor that must be considered in this present state of explosive population growth is the unevenness of the distribution among age groups. With increased medical attention to the survival and health of infants and proportionately less attention to the health of adults, the ratio between the adults—who must carry the burden of supporting and caring for children and the aged—and the children and aged means a tremendous burden on the adults; and increasing neglect of the well-being of the hordes of small children for whom there is neither proper physical provision nor an adequate number of well-trained and competent adults to care for them. The alarming increase of the death rate of men of middle age in the United States is one form that these disproportionate and excessive responsibilities take. Consider, too, the state of housing with, as an example, 35 percent of the urban population of Caracas, itself situated in the oil-rich country of Venezuela, housed in shanties on the hillsides with no visible hope of proper housing for them. It is evidenced by the tremendous number of teen-agers in the U.S.—estimated at 3 million —for whom no responsible adult can be found, if one were needed, for example, to sign a permission for surgery. These "doorstep children," uncared for, unprotected, constitute a reservoir from which a delinquent and criminal population is drawn.

Against these threatening conditions, the more locally visible effects of rapid population growth—traffic jams, parking, overcrowded schools, breakdown in services, the destruction of national parks and national monuments, the death of the trees in parks,—pale into insignificance, yet all of them decrease the well-being of the entire population, of the poor who are crowded into pollution-laden slums and of the affluent who devote so much time to commuting out of the crowded areas. No one escapes either the small, day-by-day miseries and inconveniences of overcrowding, or the larger and long-term hazards of warfare and the imminent destruction of the capacity of the planet to support the human race.

It is vitally important that the climate of opinion in regard to the value of increase of population be changed. This will involve several kinds of changes: In the economic sphere it means the abandonment of the kind of economic expansionism that demands that the gross national product grow ever greater, and that every country have a favorable balance of trade—both of which are obvious impossibilities. Exponential growth that demands exponential growth of number of consumers results in populations who can no longer be provided for except at the expense of the people of other countries, by a favorable balance of trade—which is, of course, unfavorable to other countries. If, however, nations are to abandon growth in the GNP for other indices of well-being, this will in turn involve changes in values. It is interesting that the finer things in life—human fellowship, voluntary care of other human beings, prayer, music, song and dance, love—only threaten to stress the environment when pursued in too large crowds, as at the Woodstock music festival; or the hordes of pleasure-seeking tourists who are descending upon the small and precious, delightful places in remote parts of the world where earlier generations planned and built with beauty and balance.

Specifically, governments—as policy-making instruments for the management of societies—must recognize the importance of population control. They must make massive contributions to the spread of this recognition: by a change of expansionist economic and military policies, by public measures that discourage a high birth rate, by public education through the mass media, and through example in high places. Furthermore, governmental measures will have to be supplemented by all the voluntary bodies who help to establish and maintain value systems—the churches, the schools, voluntary associations, and industry, both labor and management. Each of these institutions plays a part in the value that a society places on human well-being, on peaceful cooperation among classes and countries, upon the quality of life.

Specifically, governments, whether representative of the people or those bureaucracies that govern without a mandate from the people, can take a large number of measures conducive to population control without intruding coercively upon the choices of individual human beings. Taxes may favor small families rather than large ones, single people rather than married people, late marriage, various kinds of cooperative living rather than the ownership of expensive individual houses. Contraceptive information and equipment can be made accessible to all, with abortion as a back-up possibility where contraception fails. Legal provisions that make adoption easy and feasible are also important so that human beings, either as couples or singly, may gratify their desire to rear children without bearing them. Negative genetic counseling should be available to advise each couple who wishes to have children of the possible harmfulness of their particular genetic constitutions. Research funds should be provided to develop and test a variety of new and better contraceptive measures, as present measures prove inadequate or a danger to the long-term well-being of the population. It is especially important to pursue research also on the determination of sex so that choice of the sex of children may reduce the cost of attempting to have a child of a given sex.

The social premium we presently place upon the state of universal parenthood, with the most important pieces of information about anyone in the public eye— be he astronaut or Presidential candidate—being is he married and does he have children, should be replaced by other criteria of competence. The smallness of a given family, combined with a statement of belief in small families, should be a claim to public approval. City planning and architectural styles should provide forms of living for single and childless persons, to discourage resort to marriage and remarriage simply as necessary to ordinary daily survival and to parenthood as the only means of access to children. More community-conscious forms of living can substitute a devotion to the well-being of a group of children for the self-centered care for one's own children and grandchildren. Any attempt to attain zero population growth must recognize that it is hope for a future for children that will motivate and arouse people to the necessary long-term effort to protect lives of men, women, and children and the life of mankind.

I believe that our present information about preferences for size of family and their susceptibility to rapid change suggests that it may be possible to accomplish zero population growth without coercive governmental measures. Such measures as the introduction of contraceptive substances into a staple such as bread, or into drinking water, have been suggested, but represent such gross interference with individual liberty as to be unacceptable to any people with a democratic form of government, and possibly unfeasible even for a dictatorship type of government. Such positive interferences are repellent, but the same objections do not apply to the provision of a style of life that will tend toward small families.

It is particularly important to stress the fact that misery, poverty, hunger, and despair do not prevent population growth but in many ways promote it. The children born to the poor may be permanently injured by maternal and infant malnutrition, by the incidence of preventable disease and by the harshness of their social environment, but these conditions do not decrease and may often increase the number of children born. Having children may be the only positive and creative act left to those who eke out a miserable, deprived, and demeaned condition on insufficient welfare payments in the squalid rural slums and deteriorating ghettos. When the more affluent see children swarming in such conditions, they mistakenly infer that the children are produced in order to obtain the meager welfare benefits provided by a grudging society, instead of recognizing that it is only under conditions of less misery and more hope that people will begin to curtail the size of their families. During the splurge in population growth in the nineteen-fifties in the United States when parenthood and station wagons full of children were the style, it was the ambitious working class—anxious to get out of bad city housing—who restricted the number of their children, knowing full well that unless they did so their dream of escape would never be fulfilled. So a major contribution that a society, either locally or on a national scale, can make toward zero population growth is to combine an approved life style of small families with underwriting the kind of economic distribution that permits each human being to believe that betterment of life is possible with more effort and fewer children.

If all this is to be accomplished, if the well-being of future generations, our children, our grandchildren, our great grandchildren, is to be provided for and if this planet earth is to be saved from destruction, there are a large number of ethical considerations we must face squarely.

For those who believe in the human soul, there must be decisions about the ethicalness of refusing to give birth. Traditionally some religions have related the obligation to have children to the need to provide for reincarnation, or the obligation to welcome any of the unborn who may come to a married couple, to the need to colonize Heaven. Those who have a comfortable place on this earth have been exhorted to share their comfort by having a large number of children, and this has applied also to those well-endowed with brains, beauty, physical skill, etc. As those who carry deleterious genes are discouraged from mating, there are ethical beliefs that would encourage all those who appear to carry particularly good genes to reproduce generously. It is argued that we can only prevent the deterioration of the human species by weeding out deleterious genes and providing for the spread of desirable genes, even though at the present time, we know very little about such good genes but a great deal about the specifically deleterious ones.

These are all serious issues. The obligation to bear children, to "open the windows and let the little souls fly in," must be balanced against the right to be well-born. We have been slowly moving toward a point of view in which society will provide advocacy for the unconceived, as opposed to the previous emphasis on advocacy for the right of the conceived but not yet born. Disapproval of abortion is widespread and deep, and the arguments over the time at which an abortion should be regarded as taking a human "life" involve deep ethical feelings. It is very doubtful whether any society that made abortion into its principal public policy for population control, in preference to contraception, would fail to suffer from such a brutal solution. Elective abortion as a back-up for contraceptive failure may be justified by reference to the right of a child to be wanted and cared for, but continual resort to abortion is a brutal, wasteful, inhuman method of population control; and one—be it noted—in which women bear the brunt, in their own bodies, of the failure of a world presently managed by men to provide for adequate contraceptive measures.

Sterilization of both men and women is gaining great popularity in some countries, classes, and ethnic groups even to the advocacy of tying the tubes of women after a number of births and to bounties paid to men who will undergo vasectomies, a much less complex surgical process for males. The objections, however, are important. Such operations are for the most part irreversible and often accompanied by a sense of personal loss of adequacy and potency, both by the one who is now sterilized and by his spouse. Although the existence of sperm banks might make it possible to provide for future children, there seem at present to be rather strong arguments against sterilization measures, and every reason for making them completely personal and elective without governmental rewards of any kind. The possibility of exploitation, as when plantation workers are encouraged to undergo vasectomies so as to make them more efficient laborers who bring greater profit to their employers, or when vasectomy is promoted by a government as an alternative to attending to problems of housing, are cases in point. For the happily married man, who feels his family is complete, who can bank sperm against a change, who feels adequate in his productive role as an achieving male in contemporary society, vasectomy may become a quite satisfactory choice. These conditions are less available for the poor, and forms of population control that differ by economic class are ethically repugnant to a society committed to equal opportunity for life, liberty, and the pursuit of happiness.

Methods of contraception must also be considered in terms of fairness and equality between the sexes. No methods can be long used that permit a member of one sex to deceive the other, whether it be a male who says he has been vasectomized or a female who says that she is on The Pill, when these are lies designed for seduction by the male and for a pregnancy in a female. The ideal contraception is one that can be ascertained to be in use by both partners in a single act of sexual intercourse. Furthermore, mechanical methods that do not alter the biochemistry of the human body are to be preferred to those whose present and long-term effects are not fully known. The long-term effects of any biochemical substance cannot, in the nature of the case, be fully known until at least one generation of children born to mothers who have used The Pill have grown to reproductive age. Until such time, it should certainly be an act of choice of individuals, married pairs, and parents, as to whether The Pill, or any contraceptives of the form loosely summarized as The Pill, should be used. Certainly any compulsory or involuntary prescription should be avoided. Rumors that ghetto girls are "given" The Pill under conditions over which they have little control are almost as repulsive as the persistent rumors of involuntary sterilization of poor women at the time of delivery in a hospital. That such rumors are widespread and believed is evidence enough of the repugnance that is felt toward such interference with individual freedom of choice.

As we slowly approach a new ethical state in which the right of the unconceived replaces the right of the conceived but unborn, in our concern for individual life we may expect that advocacy of future generations' claims to consideration may become a regular part of our system of justice; and of arguments for conservation of resources, for promotion of small families where each child born will have a better chance, and for all sorts of governmental policies, for a more even distribution of national income and the devotion of a greater proportion of that income to the well-being of all of the people.

Finally, it should be pointed out that if no one who does not want a child or another child has that child, if no one who does not wish to be married is forced into marriage by current living arrangements and social pressure, if adults are permitted to live under conditions of satisfactory human companionship other than marriage, if widows and widowers are not pressured into remarriage, if adoption is facilitated, if adequate contraceptive information is available to all, and if sex determination permits parents to choose the sex of their children, this does not mean every family should have only two children. The suggested 2 and a fraction is

an average. If all of the unenthusiastic, unfit and involuntary and accidental parents were eliminated, there
would be room for some large families, those families
that do promote a kind of warmth and generosity of
character needed in any society. Those who are childless
by choice could assist in the care of large families, and it
would be possible to assure all those who wish to have at
least one child of the necessary social protection to
ensure that child adequate care, protection, and provision for a good life.

Society must be persuaded that issuing fewer invi-
tations to the next generation—one way of thinking
about the postponement of births—will make certain that
all of those invited will have a better time.

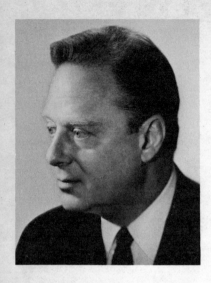

Currently the rabbi of Fairmont Temple in Cleveland, Ohio, and President of the American Jewish Congress, Arthur J. Lelyveld is also national vice-president of the American Jewish League for Israel.

During the summer of 1964, Rabbi Lelyveld went to Mississippi as a minister-counselor for the Commission on Race and Religion of the National Council of Churches. During that stay he was severely beaten by segregationists.

A member of Phi Beta Kappa, Rabbi Lelyveld received his A.B. from Columbia University in 1933. He received an M.H.L. in 1939 from Hebrew Union College, where he was ordained as Rabbi, and a degree of Doctor of Divinity from the Hebrew Union College.

Arthur J. Lelyveld

THE VISION OF OUR PLANET crawling with people "like maggots in a sack of flour"[1] is a terrifying one. Is it also an alarmist exaggeration conjured up through a too-rigid extrapolation of current rates of population growth?

The reality of Calcutta as paradigm for the comparable reality of the teeming slums in large cities East and West demonstrates the horrendous effects of too many people in too little space with too few resources.

An overcrowded planet is undeniably a possibility and it seems self-evident that the consequences of such overcrowding would be not only starvation but a scarcely imaginable kind of dehumanizing discomfort and ultimately an agonizing death.

Why, then, the debate? The nub of the controversy can be expressed in two questions:

(1) *How imminent is catastrophe?*
(2) *What are the permissible or acceptable ways of averting this catastrophe?*

A demonstratable line of causation between population growth and unavoidable human misery would lead us to expect unanimity on the necessity to limit population growth. Wherever human life is regarded as

[1] Claude Levi-Strauss.

71

supremely valuable, a commitment to its preservation must follow.

Those who pooh-pooh the predictions of ZPG advocates do so on the expectation of new and unforeseen techniques of coping with larger numbers—from farming the oceans to science-fiction-like fantasies of colonizing other planets—or on the contention that trends are reversible; and that even without controls or disasters, the birth rate frequently drops. Indeed, says one sociologist, there is also the possibility of an uncontrolled and potentially hurtful decrease in population. In the United States in 1970, even though the population of primary childbearers in the age category of twenty to twenty-four had increased by 52 percent, there were 3 million fewer children under the age of four.[2] The absence of those 3 million-plus is already being felt by schools, religious institutions, and that part of the economy that caters to children.

Others dismiss the fears of "the population controllers" as "futurology," or as a modernized version of ancient anticipations of apocalyptic catastrophe. They tell us that those who calculate a current doubling of the world population every 33 years or so and project 7 billion by the year 2,000—and 15 billion by the year 2,040—"assume there will be no major world war to kill off some of the surplus millions...."[3]

[2] George Grier, *The Baby Bust,* Washington (DC) Center for Metropolitan Studies.

[3] Rudolph Klein, *Growth and Its Enemies, Commentary* Magazine, Vol. 53 #6, June, 1972, p. 37 ff.

This grim argument offers chilling comfort: we need not worry about unchecked population growth since in one way or another we will kill each other off before we reach the saturation point. "Death control" will save us even if we fail to establish "population control."

Deprecating the warnings of those scientists who are seeking to arouse us to the dangers of continuing unchecked expansion of population and poking holes in their predictions may be an easy and inviting intellectual exercise, but it may also be self-defeating and destructive. Julian Huxley[4] reminds us that it had become customary in the early years of our century "to pooh-pooh Malthusian fear," but even though some of the particular formulations of Thomas Malthus were not correct, his general insights were well-founded and his conclusions amazingly accurate. Today's calculations buttress his assertion "that population when unchecked, increases in a geometrical progression of such a nature as to double itself every 25 years"—sometimes slower, sometimes faster, he added in a footnote—and that the means of subsistence, especially food production, increase in arithmetical progression.[5]

Thomas Malthus has been unfairly maligned, it must therefore be said. He was the first to point out a fact that has only now begun to exercise us. His limita-

---

[4] *On Population,* Three Essays: Thomas Malthus, Julian Huxley, Frederick Osborn, New American Library, New York, 1960, p. 66.
[5] Ibid, pp. 27, 29.

tion was that as a child of his time and culture he could foresee no possible positive checks other than "moral restraint, vice and misery." But he was not content that population growth would be negatively controlled by war, famine, and disease, which he saw as its inevitable results. It is the task of human institutions, he said, to diminish vice and misery, and he called for further inquiry and increased human responsibility. Even though he could recommend nothing other than "moral restraint," he opened the door for responsible, humane action, while he warned against the risk of destroying the "natural liberty" of man. In this, too, he was foreseeing the major dilemma in the issue of population control today.

The hyperboles of our latter-day Malthuses are the aspect of their preaching that turns many off. When they tell us that our grandchildren will scratch for food and crawl in their own filth, we are not so much frightened as repelled. It may be a statement of fact to say, as does Paul Ehrlich, that "In the 1970's and 1980's hundreds of millions of people will starve to death in spite of any crash programs embarked upon now";[6] but malnutrition and famine (e.g. Afghanistan, 1972) are the result of maldistribution, inadequate social planning, and sheer callousness, and would occur when these evils are present even were the birth rate to be efficiently controlled.

[6] *The Population Bomb*, Sierra Club/Ballantine, New York, 1968, p. xi.

It is also true that polemics and advocacy lead the population-control movement into the panacea fallacy. Speaking of the rise in urban violence and other evils, Ehrlich baldly affirms that "the roots of the new brutality . . . are in the lack of population control."[7] This is much too simplistic. Human depravity exists independent of human numbers. Cain murdered Abel, tribes raped and killed and looted long before there was any population problem. This is explicitly stated even by as prestigious a part of the movement as the Club of Rome's project on the predicament of mankind: ". . . Perhaps 10 to 20 million deaths each year can be attributed directly or indirectly to malnutrition. There is no question that many of these deaths are due to the world's social limitations rather than its physical ones. . . ."[8]

Another stumbling-block for the uncommitted is the special definition the movement introduces: ". . . Over-population," says Ehrlich, "does not normally mean too many people for the area of a country, but too many people in relation to the necessities and the amenities of life. Over-population occurs when numbers threaten values."[9]

This insinuates a germ of worry into our response. Whose "amenities" and whose "values"? When Frederick Osborn[10] says that "large families should be en-

[7] Ibid., p. xiii.

[8] *The Limits to Growth.* Donella H. Meadows et al. New York. Universe Books, 1972, p. 52.

[9] Op. cit., p. 9.

[10] In *On Population.* Op. cit., p. 93.

couraged for those who can maintain high standards," he suggests a kind of elitism that is disturbing even though we understand what motivates him. What high authority will make these decisions about standards? And if these exceptions are to be permitted, what will we say to those decimated culture-groups such as the Jews,who lost 6 million of their people in Hitler's "Final Solution" and who now maintain, "ZPG does not apply to us! We have the right to replenish ourselves"?

The issue of personal and group liberty is not a simple one and the dilemma is far more complex than the advocates of either extreme would lead us to believe. We can agree that a "birth-rate solution" is preferable to a "death-rate solution"; we can concur in recognizing the torture of malnutrition and that death by starvation can be a horrible process; and we can support the contention that African children doomed to kwashiorkor had better not be born—but the rub lies in the question of whether society is to determine how many children this specific couple may have or whether family planning is to be a voluntary matter, preserving the couple's right to make that determination. And when the factor of "amenity" rather than necessity is introduced, I grow concerned lest someone else decide that *my* children, or *my* grandchildren, are a threat to the quality of *his* life. This raises the specter of compulsory sterilization or contraceptive chemicals in the water supply—not so far-fetched, since both remedies have been seriously proposed.

This is why "population control" is a fighting phrase. Its advocates see it as a necessary defense against doom. To others, the word "control" suggests governmental interference in private lives and personal sanctities. There would be a much wider consensus of approval for such a phrase as "socially responsible planning for the prevention of over population."

It is the old problem of the one and the many: The precious possession of personal liberty may be in conflict with the welfare, even the survival, of society.

To put it succinctly: There is a great difference among three factors—the freedom to limit births (which I uphold); education to encourage limitation when such limitation is socially advisable (which I applaud); and compulsory limitation of births (which I fear, but which could conceivably become necessary).

Compulsory limitation would become necessary were population growth ever directly to threaten to bring about the death of others or portend the extinction of mankind. Here the Spaceship Earth analogy is pertinent. If we are all travelers on an imperiled vessel—our planet—then we are forced to agree to and submit to regulations for the good of the entire enterprise.

This analogy finds startlingly apt, proleptic support in the writings of the great Jewish physician-philosopher, Maimonides (1135-1204), who applies it in his massive Code of Jewish Law to the endorsement of abortion when the fetus threatens the life of the mother—the fetus being regarded as the pursuer or the aggressor and thus liable to destruction for the protection of the innocent pursued. Maimonides writes:

> *A boat is about to sink from the weight of its load. One passenger (with no baggage of his own) steps forward and jettisons the baggage of another to ease the boat's load. He is not liable (to make restitution), for the baggage is like a pursuer seeking to kill them; he performed a great mitzvah [fulfilled a divine command] by throwing the baggage overboard and saving the passengers.[11]*

In times of imminent danger to life—especially to the life of others—one value in the stringency of moral choice may have to be sacrificed for another and higher value. For normative Jewish thought, there is no higher value than the saving of life. In the human situation, life has supreme sanctity. Even a twentieth-century traditionalist rabbinical authority makes this absolute statement. "There is nothing that stands in the way of saving life."[12] The context in which this statement is made is a discussion of permission to take contraceptive action in an individual case—but by extension, it may be applied *a fortiori* to the problem of society.

[11] *Yad, Hovel U'Mazzik.* 8, 15 cited in David M. Feldman, *Birth Control in Jewish Law,* New York University Press, 1968, p. 278.
[12] Cited in Feldman, op. cit., p. 203.

It must be stressed that in rabbinic thought both the intent of the act and the method used are of decisive importance. The command, "Be fruitful and multiply and fill the earth" (Genesis I:28; compare Genesis IX-1, 7 and Genesis XXV:11) was given so that man will not neglect the *preservation* of the world in its human frame of reference. But equally high value is given to the joy of the marital relationship, the fulfillment of the wife's conjugal rights, and the protection of both parties against physical hazard. The joy is not of secondary importance. "He whose intent is for pleasure, does not sin," says Rabbi Isaiah da Trani.[13] Thus, even in orthodox Jewish thought, the use of intrauterine devices or of birth-control pills seems to be unimpeachable if the intent is correct.

This has direct bearing on the line between "amenity" and "necessity." We must ask how lethal the threat is, and know that only a threat that is demonstratedly lethal would warrant any interference with personal liberty. "Precaution against physical hazard is a *mitzvah*; as to financial exigency, the very idea of allowing it to figure in considerations of birth-control seems unworthy," Rabbi David Feldman concludes.[14]

What is stressed by rabbinic tradition is the obligation for reasonable and responsible habitation of the world; and one can deduce from the fact that contra-

---

[13] Feldman, op. cit., p. 162, cf. p. 105.
[14] Op. cit., p. 303.

ception is permitted to nursing mothers for the sake of the welfare of *existing* children that we, as a society, have an obligation to be provident with respect to the welfare of *existing* human beings. Certainly, then, there is a relationship between this attitude toward birth control and the societal implications of the dire, if conditional, prediction of 33 leading scientists:

> *If current trends are allowed to persist, the break-down of society and the irreversible disruption of the life-support systems on this planet—possibly by the end of the century, certainly within the lifetimes of our children—are inevitable.*[15]

The halcyon picture of Psalm 128 is a normal aspiration in human life: "Thy wife shall be as a fruitful vine . . . thy children like olive plants around thy table." But this male-oriented dream of blessedness has to be balanced against the personal aspirations of the wife and her own right to personal fulfillment as a human being in ways that she herself shall choose, and against the needs of humankind when the olive plants threaten to strangle themselves and to erase the implied bliss of the scene through malign overgrowth.

The task is to define our crises—ecological and demographic—soberly and accurately, and then to or-

[15] From "Blueprint for Survival" in *The Ecologist* Magazine. See *N.Y. Times,* January 14, 1972.

ganize ourselves, nationally and globally, to take necessary action, with as effective protection of the values of
personal liberty and human fulfillment as the crisis will
permit. In this Frederick Osborn is correct when he says
that we must not assume that religious loyalties, East or
West, will be a major obstacle to the changes that are
determined upon as necessary. Indeed, because of the
social and ethical considerations that lie compellingly
behind the population-control movement, the religions
themselves may be vehicles for its realization.[16] There
can be no "sanctification of life" in the suicide of the
human race. Indeed, preserving life, and preserving its
humane potentialities, is essentially what we mean by
sanctifying life, filling the world with the presence of the
Divine.

The religions, therefore, will undoubtedly play a
major role in supporting the United Nations effort to
concentrate on this problem, with 1974 now named
World Population Year as a target date for the needed
studies and surveys to compile statistics, population-
growth estimates, and information on the various aspects
of fertility and family planning in every nation, as well
as globally. This is a belated response to the plea U
Thant made in 1969 to the members of the UN "to sub-
ordinate their ancient quarrels and launch a global
partnership to curb the arms race, to defuse the population explosion and to supply the required momentum to

[16] *On Population,* op. cit., p. 107.

development efforts. . . ."[17]

There is a quaint rabbinical parable that tells of three men in a boat, two of whom are horrified when they see the third take an auger and bit and calmly begin to drill a hole in the bottom. When they wildly protest, he, in effect, tells them to cool it and says, "What's it to you? I'm just drilling under my own seat!"

Before it is utterly too late, and with full regard for *all* of our sanctities, we must come to realize that we are all—all of us on Spaceship Earth—in the same boat.

[17] See *The Limits to Growth*. Op. cit., proem.

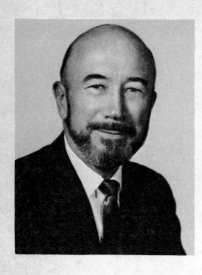

Dr. Preston Cloud, Professor of Biogeology at the University of California, knows the resources of our earth as few others do. Dr. Cloud served for many years as geologist for the U. S. Geological Survey, and has been member and chairman of various Congressional panels on resources and population problems.

He is especially interested in the development of new insights into the future of expanding man on a finite earth, and for his work in this vital area, has received such awards as the Rockefeller Public Service Award, the Distiniguished Service Award and Medal of the U. S. Department of the Interior, and the A. Cressy Morrison Prize of the New York Academy of Sciences.

Dr. Cloud is also editor and co-author of two important books, RESOURCES AND MAN and ADVENTURES IN EARTH HISTORY, and has published many technical books and articles in the field of his specialization.

Preston Cloud

IT IS HARD TO IMAGINE or even to accept something you have not seen—the agony of Bangladesh, the favelae of Brazil, the general condition of life in India, the slums of Western cities as you pass over them on the freeway, or even the 75 million additional mouths to feed that appeared on earth last year. It has also been hard, until recently, for man to grasp the concept of a limited earth. Those pictures of earth taken from the Apollo space-craft have finally done what words had been unable to do. They have created a broad, if not universal, aware-ness of the finiteness and delicacy of our planet.

When will we put this together with the often-repeated and staggering statistics of exponential popula-tion growth to realize that, unless we do something about it, an irresistible force is about to meet an immov-able object?

It is the *rates* of growth in population and demand that have suddenly brought about this dilemma—not to say, crisis. These rates, like compound interest on a loan, cause the thing multiplied to double over a period of time; and, like interest rates, they have been increasing. The 250 million or so people on earth at the time of Christ took 1,650 years to reach 500 million, but the second doubling occurred in two hundred years, the third in eighty years, and the fourth, to 4 billion, expected by about 1975, will take only about forty-five years. *Present* rates of population increase, if continued, will lead to doubling times of about thirty-five years for the world as a whole and seventy years for its now-affluent parts. As most of the people now on earth are too young to have yet had children of their own, there is also a built-in momentum to population growth that makes future increases inevitable, assuming no global catastrophe.

We are now barely able to manage a world population of 3.8 billion and a U.S. population of 208 million. How shall we feed, house, transport, and amuse the 6 to 7 billion earthians and 280 million or so Americans expected by the year 2,000, let alone improve on today's preponderantly miserable levels of living? Indeed, how shall we care for the 5.7 billion earthians and 286 million Americans to be expected no later than 2,042, even at bare replacement rates of 2.1 children per couple for those who have not yet had their families? And, if we agree that these numbers must not be exceeded, what steps should we take to avert that?

These are hard questions. The answers to them vary widely, depending on personal viewpoints, not only about what the facts mean, but also about such things as upward mobility, the state of the economy, the sufficiency of resources, the potency of technology, the environmental consequences of growth, personal freedom, and the dignity of man.

Economists and demographers have worried about

the social and economic trade-offs. Immediate attainment of ZPG would mean prompt retrenchment to the one-child family as a universal norm, with severe social and economic repercussions. Within a generation populations would become as top-heavy at the upper end of the age spectrum as they now are at the lower end. The present generation of young people would become the only one in history to outnumber both its predecessors and its successors, and would be likely to dominate and repress the latter accordingly. Upward job mobility would be limited and age at retirement would need to be lowered drastically (not a bad idea) if unemployment were not to soar. Economic growth would slow down or stop. And matters would be even "worse" in the overdeveloped countries if their levels of affluence were restrained (as they should be) in order to reduce environmental impact and permit the now-deprived to catch up.

Although ZPG and a steady state economy are both inevitable consequences on a finite earth, I am persuaded by these arguments to believe that it is unrealistic to hope for anything more drastic than an early acceptance of the two-child mode. Even without the economists and a few old-fashioned demographers to warn us, my limited grasp of human perceptions and responses suggests that even this is going to take some doing.

On the other hand, there are some encouraging signs. For generations it was regarded as obscene to write about or discuss birth control, and people were jailed for exhibiting or even for using birth-control devices. But suddenly, only a little over a decade ago, it became acceptable not only to discuss openly but to practice birth control, as well as to assist other nations with "family planning" programs. Even abortion is now openly advocated and practiced, although by no means widely enough. The simple fact that we have moved rather quickly from this to open discussion of population *control*, therefore, offers hope that the concept may be more widely accepted in the affluent world than its "leaders" recognize. If they want to stay leaders, and not of beggar nations, it is time for them to get in front and do what they can to reduce the perils of runaway populations—first by proclamation of population control as a national and global goal and then by all means of public persuasion compatible with free societies.

What can they do? They can stop talking about "family planning to help everybody have the size family he wants," and emphasize that continuing population growth poses serious hazards to the welfare of present and future generations alike. They can stop extolling the virtues of ever-increasing material growth and per capita rates of consumption and point with alarm to the multiplying effects this has on consumption of resources and degradation of the ecosystem, and thus on the austerity that future generations may face. They can encourage attitudes, pass laws, and establish regulations that will have restraining effects on population growth, in order that the other and more important freedoms than unrestrained procreation may be preserved. They can admit and take steps to deal with the difficulties likely to be caused by essential restraining measures, while stressing that the latter are demanded by an enlightened view of our own welfare and a humane consideration for the rights and needs of the unborn.

Daniel Callahan expressed it well in a recent article, "Ethics and Population Limitation" (*Science*, February, 1972), when he wrote:

> *Since individuals are obliged to respect the rights of others, they are obliged to act in such a way that these rights are not jeopardized. In determining family size, this means that they must exercise their own freedom of choice in such a way that they do not curtail the freedom of others. They are obliged, in short, to respect the requirements of the common good in their exercise of free choice.*

There is even a good deal of unwarranted confusion about what the facts are. A front-page headline in the *San Francisco Chronicle* recently (February 17, 1972) proclaimed, "U.S. Approaching Zero Growth in Population," a conclusion it derived from a Census Bureau report that "the average number of children *expected* [italics mine] by wives aged eighteen to twenty-four plummeted from 2.9 to 2.4." Even if the actual fertility rate fell to 2.2 children as the *Chronicle* suggests, that approaches not a zero rate of growth but a simple "replacement rate." A bare replacement rate, as pointed out above, will not lead to ZPG before the year 2,042, even if begun now and maintained until then—at which time the U.S. population would be 286 million. Leaving out the occasional dips in general fertility rates that bring out fearful cries of dropping populations from those who thrive on population increases, the projected trend—taking all actual and potential reproductive groups in this country into consideration—is still an increase of barely under 1 percent per year, which, if continued, gives a doubling time of about seventy-two years. I applaud the ladies for the trend in their goals, but those goals must decline still further; and *unexpected* births must be eliminated, before the nation will reach even bare replacement levels of reproduction. And we can ill stress to the deprived world its desperate need for ZPG if we hold a lesser goal for ourselves.

Going back to individual freedom, my view is that it is hard to overdo. I subscribe completely to the declaration of the *1968 United Nations International Conference on Human Rights* that "couples have a basic human right to decide freely *and responsibly* [italics mine] on the number and spacing of their children and a right to adequate information and education in this respect." If individual decisions are, in fact, to be responsible, of course, education in this context must include not only the basic techniques of fertility control, but also the likely consequences of continued population growth.

Consider the capacity of earth to support people. The Committee on Resources and Man of the National Academy of Sciences of the U.S. made some estimates of earth's limits in 1969. They concluded that a *maximum* of about 30 billion could be fed at a general level comparable to that now found in India, but that the world would be hard-pressed to support even 7 billion at levels of affluence comparable to those in the United States. Continuation of present doubling rates would bring world population to around 7 billion by the end of the century and 30 billion in about a hundred years. Thus, there is no time to waste in inquiring how populations may be limited to levels that best assure the eventual attainment of a life of high quality for all men everywhere, including a wide flexibility and freedom of choices in matters other than size of family.

Indeed, it is now generally conceded by informed demographers, ecologists, and students of natural resources that a zero or negative rate of population growth is eventually inevitable on a finite earth. The question is no longer whether ZPG is desirable or not, but how and when it will take place, at what rate, and with what consequences. Will it take place because thoughtful and responsible people prefer it, or when the limitations of earth are discovered the hard way and population growth is terminated by war, famine, pestilence, deterioration of the human spirit, or some combination of these things? For it is an immutable law of nature that disturbance of any balanced state is always followed by reactions that tend to restore the balance.

Promotion of attitudes, mores, and suitable incentive legislation that will move norms toward smaller family sizes and modes of personal fulfillment that do not involve parenthood can take place in many directions. First steps should include universal legal abortion, free on request to the indigent and inexpensive for others; universally accessible free birth-control clinics; rewriting of first-readers to show more happy maiden aunts and bachelors, with less emphasis on family life as the fulfillment norm; legalization of homosexual relations between consenting adults; and revision of current tax laws and welfare regulations to discourage parenthood without depriving children of amenities and opportunities. In my view, also, the world situation is sufficiently ominous that we should both increase nonmilitary foreign aid and reassess the conditions under which it is given to encourage attitudes that favor self-help and limitation of populations. Many and touching though the arguments against any limitations are, it is of little value to deplete the earth and strain its resilience merely in order that larger populations may live in even greater misery and die more prematurely later on.

Growth of populations affects people in many ways. Our blighted cities, our besieged universities, our deteriorating resource base, our vanishing wilderness, our overregulated lives, and our threatened ecosystem in general are all, in some sense, a consequence of excessive numbers and demands. Two thirds of the world even now live under conditions of undernourishment and privation. The other third will face its own agonizing problems: What to do about the pressures on its gates by the less privileged? How to cope with the increasing burden of biocides, nuclear wastes, mine wastes, air and water pollution, and noise? How to endure the necessary increase of regulatory measures (and taxes) flowing from competition for resources, space, recreation, transportation, housing, educational facilities, and privacy?

The preservation of freedom from the excessive regulation of life, of flexibility of options for the future, of general environmental quality, of wilderness and other open space, of safeguards against excessive loss of life and property from natural catastrophes does not come free. It can be gained only at the cost of an earlier reduction than might otherwise be necessary of economic growth and eventually of a steady state economy, of nonincrease or reduced rates of increase of property "values," of some limitation of upward mobility and career advancement, and, above all, of population growth.

I find no difficulty in choosing between these alternatives for myself or my descendants, and I have little doubt that this choice would become a majority view if all could appreciate how closely we press on the limits of our planet to support all of its human passengers and a decent variety of other life at a quality level. Look at some purely local growth-related problems. Is it right for the San Francisco urban region to grow more populous where that means building more dwelling places along the San Andreas fault or on the unstable bayheads flats, where they will shake apart in the next major earthquake? Is it right for Los Angeles realtors or others to prosper on high-rise or hillside construction that constitutes an open invitation to earthquake damage, foundation failure, and other hazards? Is it right for industrial Buffalo to pollute the atmosphere of rural upstate New York or for Washington, D.C., to foul the Potomac? As urbanization spreads over hazard-prone areas that should be reserved for green belts, more and more such places are likely to become temporary disaster areas for avoidable reasons. Many potential hazards would be greatly reduced or would not exist were human populations not so large; or were they better distributed; or were consumption and waste disposal reduced and better managed. In most instances, new and costly regional enviromental authorities, new and thoughtful incentive legislation, and Federal and regional initiatives will be required. They will be needed to see that the things we already know are applied to improve the present situation and prevent a worsening in the future.

They will be needed to generate the research and development that is essential for better understanding of our total ecosystem and resource base. And they will be needed to assure the continuing overview and early warning systems that alone (and to limited degree) can safeguard the integrity and sufficiency of our environment against the consequences of increasing concentrations of people.

Human response to official declaration and actions being unpredictable and often perverse, there is no telling what it might be to an explicit proclamation of population control as a national or global goal. The issues are critical enough, however, that it is worth trying to aid their resolution by public statements of goals; by appropriation of funds for research, development, and education leading toward better understanding and management of environment, resources, and populations; and by imaginative incentive and enabling legislation. Even where beneficial goals and desired norms are generally accepted, behavior that will lead to their attainment often lags where the indifferent, the callous, or the slovenly are not nudged into constructive directions by some code that helps the responsible citizen to follow the dictates of his conscience without penalty and encourages the indifferent one to shape up. To be effective, such a code must involve appropriate legal frameworks.

For ten thousand or more years the aboriginal inhabitants of the United States, never greater in number than three million, lived generally in harmony and balance with nature. In a little over three hundred years—and especially in the last hundred—a new nation of immigrants, with economic growth and the conquest of nature as its code and material possessions its measure of achievement, has multiplied 170 times, filled the continent, bent nature to its will, and amassed material things. Two hundred eight million people of our style of life, movement, and consumption, with all their stunning achievements and bright potentialities, already press hard on the capacity of the continent to supply fresh water, clean air, and ample open space for urban vacationists. They exceed its limits in their demands for mineral raw materials, a large fraction of which now come from foreign sources. As a student of earth history, I cannot help wondering whether this nation will last as long as the Indians it displaced. I wonder whether man will last as long as the species he has exterminated. I believe that whether he does or not will depend very much on the degree to which we now apprehend the problems, and on what we do over the next two or three decades to limit human populations and strike a new balance with nature, here and abroad. Contrary to the views of some, and despite the hysteria that clouds its calm and rational perception, I share the conviction expressed by Robert McNamara in his 1970 address to the Board of Governors of the World Bank Group—namely that the prospect for man's future is a matter of grave and immediate concern in which the key issue is population control.

To return to the question of human rights, I hold that the above and other evidence makes it essential to recognize two new fundamental human rights:

1. *The right of the fetus not to be conceived, or if conceived, not born, into a world where its existence is likely to be precarious, to threaten the security of its siblings, or to increase the hazard to the general welfare.* It strikes me as in some deep sense uncivilized, not to say irresponsible, to consider babies as objects without rights, that people are entitled to propagate at will regardless of the kind of life the growing child and later adult is likely to live, or regardless of the general welfare. Instead, the rights of the unborn or unconceived, who have neither foresight nor judgment, should take precedence, if necessary, over those of adults, who are at least capable of foreseeing the consequences of their actions. Above all, no woman should be forced to carry an unwanted child to term. To those who speak of the fetus as a person, I ask what reasonable concept of freedom can condone the "right" of one person to live *in* the body of another against that other's will? Compulsory pregnancy, at any stage, should be abolished as the barbaric and unconstitutional practice it is.

2. *The right of society as a whole, through democratic processes, to influence the sizes of populations in ways and directions that best assure a continuing flexibilty of options,* including access to such resources of food, clean air, and water, essential raw materials, and space as best assure a meaningful existence.

But what if education, persuasion, tax incentives,

and other noncoercive or only mildly coercive measures don't produce the desired response? Should governments then take more direct action to limit birth and populations, as they habitually claim the right to do in other areas of behavior (*e.g.* marriage) affecting the general welfare? If so, should such measures apply equally to wealthy and poor, to the educated and uneducated, to "good" and "bad" parents alike? And how should religious or moral convictions be handled?

These are hard questions that we may all hope need never be answered, but which we should think about beforehand in case the need to answer them arises. If education, persuasion, and tax incentives were to bring about public responses that led to the two-child family as the norm, the number of childless women and one-child families would compensate for reasonable numbers of three- or even four-child families. There is some, if small, reason in past responses and present concerns to hope that this may lead to volutary population control, at least in the affluent world. The developing world is another problem. Tradition, personal prestige, social security, and religious conviction all contribute importantly (together with ignorance, nonavailability of means, and medical reduction of infant deaths) to the inertial effects that keep the population explosion going strong in these countries. So do the recurring proclamations of "planned parenthood" agencies that the problem is about to go away because births per thousand have dropped from forty to thirty-five per year (the

"stable" level is fourteen per thousand at a seventy-year
life expectancy).

If I were to grasp the nettle, I would say that, should
voluntary measures not show good prospects of moving
toward balanced populations within another decade,
stronger measures should be seriously and democratically considered. Of course, if the majority elects to find
the limits the hard way, there will be little to do about
it that is acceptable in any democratic and open sense.
But it is not impossible that public support might be
mustered for some open and equitable system of limitations. A number of such systems have been suggested and
probably will be suggested by others in this book. And
Daniel Callahan, in the paper mentioned earlier, enum-
erates general criteria for choosing which system is
likely to do least violence to concepts of human dignity
and individual freedom, as well as some of the difficulties, costs, and unpleasant consequences of trying to
enforce any coercive system.

If, after due trial of voluntary methods, such a
system should appear essential for survival and the
preservation of other freedoms, it must above all be
equitable. Apart from grounds of human dignity and
individual rights, we must remember that man is an
evolving creature on an evolving earth. His greatest
asset in meeting future opportunities and changes is a
heterogeneous gene pool. Genius and idiocy appear about
as frequently among the children of the deprived and
unschooled as they do among those of the prosperous

and the educated. The acquisition of wealth, education, or social status by parents offers no assurance that their children will be better able to cope with the real world. Indeed, the reverse may be true.

The time to establish favorable terms with nature through our own conscious and thoughtful action is short and growing shorter. Real population control, in the sense that national and world populations are caused to stabilize at reasonable levels within reasonable time, is essential to the future well-being and dignity of man and the preservation of more important freedoms than the right to procreate.

After all, it is not such a large step from regulating the number of wives or husbands a person may have to regulating the number of children, and a great deal more is at stake.

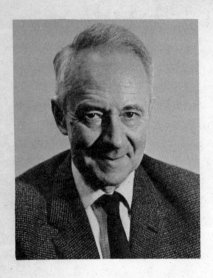

British agricultural economist Colin Grant Clark is the author of POPULATION GROWTH AND LAND USE: STARVATION OR PLENTY, CONDITIONS OF ECONOMIC PROGRESS, THE ECONOMICS OF SUBSISTENCE AGRICULTURE, THE ECONOMICS OF IRRIGATION, *and a number of other topical and significant books.*

Dr. Clark is a member of the French Academy of Agriculture, and a Fellow and former Council Member of both the Econometric Society and the Royal Statistical Society. He is on the faculty of Monash University.

He holds honorary degrees from the universities of Milan and Tilburg, and until 1969, was director of the Agricultural Economics Institute at Oxford University.

Colin Clark

THE UNITED STATES was founded upon a passionate belief in the rights of man. "Life, liberty, and the pursuit of happiness" was an abbreviated expression, adumbrated more thoroughly by social philosophers, ancient and modern. The rights of man include the right to express himself on matters of political and public concern, the right to form associations, the rights to own property and do business, and the right to marry and bring up a family. These rights are widely violated in the present-day world—just as they were in the past by American and other slave owners. In most countries in the world now, the people are forbidden to express themselves on politics; and in many of them, they are not allowed to carry on their own businesses either. The denial of the right to family life was probably the most hideous aspect of slavery; and also of the racial repression in South Africa and Rhodesia, where men are forcibly separated from their families by the work and residence permit systems.

But what are the qualifications to these natural rights of man? It is sometimes said that they cease to be valid if they do harm to others. This will not do at all. Your business may do harm to mine by successfully competing with me. This certainly does not give me the right to demand that your business should be closed down. The rights of man are only limited if they are used to perform actual injustice against others. The right of political free speech is limited if a man speaks defamation against individuals, contempt against judges, or sedition against his government. The rights of owning property and forming associations must not be used to exact extortionate terms from weaker parties.

And the right of establishing and bringing up a family?

If you tell another man that you propose to stop him bringing up a family because you find the consequences inconvenient, you are completely unjustified. Suppose, however, you could prove that the birth and upbringing of his children was inflicting real injustice on you, for example reducing you and your family to near-starvation. Even in this highly theoretical case it would be very difficult to prove that you were entitled to compel him to limit his family. Even people starving under siege conditions have tried to do the best they could for newborn children. In fact, as evidence from all over the world shows, when threatened with actual famine, parents themselves are most unlikely to conceive. The man who claims the right compulsorily to limit other people's families will have to prove that his country is threatened with permanent, not with temporary famine, and that other people have become so improvident that they completely fail to recognize this.

The whole case is a non-starter. So, far from being threatened with famine, we are threatened with an embarrassing overabundance of food. Even the lesser case, that population growth causes inconvenience, cannot be substantiated. So, far from being a disadvantage, population growth brings greater advantages—economic, political, and cultural—in the United States and in other countries. Proposals for the compulsory limitation of families, which would be an infringement of the rights of man in any case, are also based on misinformation about the facts.

How so many people in the United States—and to some extent in other countries, too—otherwise intelligent and well-informed, are so hysterically denouncing population growth, when all the facts show its effects to be favorable, is a question that only a social psychologist can answer. To an outside observer, it appears that the United States now, particularly the younger generation, is in a positive frenzy of self-hatred, almost deserving the psychologists' phrase "death wish." For those who roundly condemn American civilization in all its forms, it is perhaps consistent to go on and conclude that the fewer Americans the better.

But there is more to it than this. Those who are deeply committed to family limitation in their own personal lives tend to develop extremely strong feelings (possibly based upon envy) that other people ought to limit their families, too; and that if they do not do so voluntarily, they ought to be compelled.

In this, as in many other doctrines now circulating among the younger educated men and women, there is a strong element of "elitism." We are the elite, they feel strongly, and we do not want the lower classes to outnumber us. There is a strong element of concealed racial prejudice in this attitude, too. It is well-known that the colored races, in the United States and elsewhere, and peasant communities throughout the world are multiplying much more rapidly than those living in the advanced civilizations. This, they feel, ought to be stopped. But how unrealistic is their outlook? Even if they succeeded in passing legislation in the United States for compulsory sterilization of poor black families (what a hope!) nothing that is done in the United States or Western Europe will reduce family size in Asia, Africa, or Latin America. In fact, our antics may encourage them to further population growth—for reasons that we may find ominous.

So the case for compulsory limitation of families is knocked out in a few paragraphs. It would be a flagrant denial of the rights of man. But, quite apart from this issue, this proposal is based on misinformation about the facts. The remainder of this text will be devoted to showing that population growth is advantageous in every respect.

While most people are concerned with the economic consequences (which they believe to be harmful) of population growth, it has political and cultural consequences, too. These, if less easy to measure, are in some ways more important; and we may consider them first.

The United States has enjoyed continuous population growth ever since the Pilgrim Fathers landed in 1620. Because it is so much a part of the American background, few people have ever stopped to analyze its effects. But they have been all-pervading. There is scarcely any aspect of American life—economic, political, or cultural—which would have developed as it has, had it not been for population growth.

As an alternative, we are, of course, not discussing what would have happened had the country remained virtually uninhabited. But suppose that the Americans at some comparatively early date had decided to check population growth by limiting immigration and by reducing the size of their families. Both of these measures were taken in the 1920s. But by that time, the United States had well over 100 million population, and the course of development was already well set. Had population limitation been initiated at an early date, one of the first consequences would probably have been that what is now the United States would not have been an English-speaking community at all, but French-speaking or Spanish-speaking.

The situation can be seen more clearly from the other side of the fence. The French demographer Sauvy points out as something quite obvious that the reason why the greater part of North America became English-speaking was demographic, namely that the British Isles, from the mid-eighteenth century onward, had higher rates of natural increase of population than the rest of Europe, and could, therefore, supply more immigrants. He might have added that the early settlers were not only willing to bring up large families, but also lived healthy and hygienic lives, and suffered comparatively low mortality rates by the standards of the time; and so their own rate of natural increase was the highest in the world.

Whether we like it or not, there is an unavoidable connection between population and world power status.

It will be useful to begin by examining in detail a few obvious propositions. The United States is a world power. What precisely do we mean by this? We mean that statesmen all over the world, planning their countries' foreign policies, have to take into account what the United States may think or do; indeed further, that the United States is in a position to influence, by methods ranging from tactful suggestions to open threats, events anywhere in the world. It is, of course, by no means implied that it is either wise or expedient for the United States always so to intervene; or that past decisions to intervene, or not to intervene, have always been soundly judged. In this sense, it is clear, the United States is a world power, and Mexico is not—important though Mexico's foreign policy decisions may be to her immediate neighbors.

It is another well-known fact that the United States now has a population of 210 million and Mexico 54 million. The facts of world power and of population are inescapably connected. Americans sometimes like to think that it is their advanced industrial technology, rather than the size of their population, that makes them a world power. Switzerland has an industrial technology comparable with that of the United States; Soviet Russia, comparable with that of Mexico. Soviet Russia is a world power, and Switzerland is not. Some people have yielded to the superficial theory that in these days of nuclear and other advanced weaponry, size of population has ceased to matter. Indeed, it probably matters more than before, as historical comparisons will show. The technical ability to produce advanced weapons is only one element in a country's ability to become a world power. Equally necessary are the very large economic resources needed to produce and maintain them. The size of a country's population also plays an important part in its ability to exert economic, political, or cultural influence in the world; or indeed, to construct adequate defenses or retaliatory measures against nuclear warfare, or—if the worst comes to the worst— to recover from its consequences.

A few centuries ago, England had a population of only 6 million, as against France's 20 million. But two much smaller countries, Netherlands and Sweden, with a population of only a little over a million each, were then respectively the greatest naval and military powers in Europe. They both had established settlements in North America, and were well-set in the race for possession. It was only a military alliance between the English and the French, albeit temporary, that drove the Dutch out of New York.

It was possible for countries of very small population to become world powers in those days, precisely because military and naval equipment was very simple and cheap; and so also, indeed, were mercenary soldiers. The Dutch Army at that time consisted largely of foreign volunteers who were attracted in sufficient numbers by the pay of six pence per day. Countries that were economically a little ahead of their neighbors, as Netherlands and Sweden were then, could thereby become world powers.

A century later, mercenary soldiers—though higher paid—were less effective, as the British generals found in the American war. The new world power of those days was Prussia, with a population of 6 million, much below Austria and France. But observe that the minimum population required by a country that was to be a world power was six times what it had been a century earlier.

In the 1870s, Great Britain was still the leading world power—though this was largely due to the accidental circumstances that the two principal potential rivals, United States and France, had both been temporarily devastated by war. Britain's population at that time was 31 million. A newly emerging world power was Italy, with a population of 27 million—again more than a four-fold increase on the minimum population required a century earlier.

We are at this time prepared to look at the 1970s. The number of great world powers is indeed shrinking. The only countries that really matter now in world politics are the United States, Russia, China, India, and perhaps Japan—the latter with a population of 105 million, again four times the minimum required a century earlier. Indonesia, with a population of 125 million, may conceivably become a world power at a later date, but .has immense economic and political difficulties to overcome.

There is no escaping the conclusion that world power is becoming concentrated more—not less—in the hands of the countries with large populations.

If population does not grow by natural increase or by migration, there is a third way, namely by amalgamation. The former world powers of Western Europe—with their slowly growing populations—becoming aware of their rapidly diminishing importance in the world scene, have formed an economic union among themselves, which will probably soon ripen into a full political union, which will again be a power in the world. In view of Europe's political maturity, and the sad experience of her own nationalistic excesses in the past, it may well be hoped that such a European union will become a powerful force for world peace.

Similar unions may perhaps be formed in Latin America, in Africa, and in Southeast Asia, with the prospect also of becoming world powers. But these possibilities are remote.

So much for the grim world power game. In the past, even as late as 1941, many Americans thought that it was possible, while being militarily prepared, to stay outside the world power game. Nobody thinks that way any more. In the world as it is now, a country that remains isolated without allies, however large and powerful, runs the risk of subjugation.

From this harsh but necessary topic, we may turn to the relationship between population growth and freedom. Even people who are satisfied that the world can yield the economic resources to provide for a larger population are concerned lest population growth mean a loss of freedom, and that the increased populations of the future will have to lead strictly regulated lives.

The opposite is the case. In the face of the evidence, the proposition is not a very sensible one. After all, the world has acquired what freedoms it has in the course of the last two or three centuries of rapid population growth, not in the long centuries of stationary or very slowly growing population that preceded them.

The same is true of economic freedom. Though still subject to imperfections, the United States has shown the world how to develop a highly productive economic system based on free competition, with agreements among businessmen to fix prices and divide markets treated as a punishable offense. Now to take an extreme example, Governor Bradford, administering the hungry pioneer settlement of the Pilgrim Fathers, could not have introduced a competitive economic system, however much he had wanted to. Free competition is capable of conferring great benefits on the world; but it can only work under certain specified circumstances. To take another example, the medieval towns, though they represented a considerable advance, alike in economic productivity and in political freedom, over the rural manors cultivated by serfs who surrounded them, nevertheless lived under a system of regulated prices, and cartels or guilds of craftsmen designed to exclude competition. They could not do otherwise. Other towns, with which they could have entered into more productive and competitive economic relationships, were some distance away; and transport and communications were excessively costly and often dangerous. Even in the modern world with its almost infinitely better transport and communications, neither a competitive economy nor a free political system are found to work well in small isolated islands, which always tend to come under the domination of powerful interests.

A stationary population, so far from making the world freer, would greatly increase the amount of government regulation required. This is illustrated by the writings of Lord Keynes. Keynes (whom I knew well) was certainly the most remarkable economist of his time, not least in his capacity to change his mind. In 1926, he published a book which had a great deal of influence, *The End of Laissez Faire*. Laissez faire was the phrase then used for a free competitive economy. Keynes contended, on quite strong evidence, that this had only been possible under the conditions of growing population that had prevailed in the nineteenth century.

With the prospect of population growth ceasing altogether (so it appeared to the thinkers in the 1920s), laissez faire would have to be abandoned, and government regulation of investment take its place. A stationary population, Keynes said, could not stand the mistakes in investment that private business would make, and he thought (at that time) that government investment would be better planned.

But by 1937, Keynes, still following the same line of reasoning, had reached a very different conclusion. By then, he had lost his faith in the wisdom of government investment policies, and wanted to restore a world in which the main investment decisions were made by private business. But this would only be possible, he rightly pointed out, when population growth—which had indeed much slowed down in the 1930s—once again resumed.

This point was stated still more forcefully in recent years by Professor Everett Hagen, of the Massachusetts Institute of Technology. Population growth, to use his striking phrase, "absolves" a country from the consequences of errors in investment, whether by private business or by governments. With a stationary population, an erroneous investment is likely to be a dead loss. But with a growing population, some use is likely to be found before long for the misplaced investment.

In the '30s, when it appeared for a time not only that population growth had stopped, but that an actual decline was likely to set in, there were indeed some strange ideas expressed. Lord Stamp, the leading British orthodox economist of those days (Keynes being the leading heterodox), chairman of the largest private railway company, a director of the Bank of England, and one of the Government's principal advisers, in his capacity as president of the British Association for the Advancement of Science, propounded in 1936 that now that population was stationary, technical progress was proceeding too fast; and solemnly advanced the proposal that a tax ought to be imposed upon technical innovations, in order to give the old equipment time to wear out and men with the old skills time to retire. "Birth control for people necessitates birth control for their impedimenta" was his curious summary.

In France, where population had been stationary for a considerably longer period, the situation was worse. As Louis Armand, a leading administrator, has pointed out, Malthusianism created *le malthusianisme economique*, with every kind of restrictive practice, discouragement of innovation, and technical backwardness.

The relation of population growth to culture is more difficult to measure. On a question like this, we must press into service all the evidence that we can obtain from history, because at best the number of examples is limited.

However, we are in a position to draw some conclusions for the reason that until recently sustained population growth was quite a rare event in the history of the world; and when it does occur, we are in a position to isolate and examine its consequences. These are nearly always seen to be great advances alike in the economic, political, and cultural fields. There is a reason why this should be so. If we adopt the theory (for which there is a good deal of evidence) that the majority of men are inherently lazy and unprogressive, and only make changes when compelled by population growth or some similar overwhelming pressure, then many of the observed facts can be explained.

Of the periods of rapid population growth within a limited land area, the first of which we have record is that of the ancient Greeks in the sixth and fifth centuries B.C. Their writers were constantly complaining about poverty and shortage of land. But we all know that, in response to this challenge, they created what is still regarded as the finest civilization the world has ever seen, with great achievements in art, literature, science, and philosophy. From their small base, they spread flourishing colonies all over the Mediterranean and Black Sea, settling as far as Marseilles and the Crimea. Economically, they converted their tribal and agricultural society into a productive manufacturing economy—within the limits of the technology of those days, but probably as productive as that of nineteenth-century Europe—with widespread international commerce. And politically, they rendered the world the inestimable service of pioneering democratic forms of government.

After this comes a long interval until the early Middle Ages, from the eleventh to thirteenth centuries,

which are known to have been a period of rapid population growth. With this came another great flowering
of civilization, centered in France and Italy. Though not
a free society by our standards, it was certainly a great
improvement, both economically and politically, on that
of the preceding centuries.

The Dutch in the sixteenth century were a small and
vigorous people whose growing numbers were cooped
up on a few inhospitable mudbanks. There are few
events in history so astonishing as their rapid rise to become the leading commercial, colonizing, and naval
power of the world, founding New York, Capetown, and'
Djakarta all within a single decade. With no motive
power other than men, horses, and windmills, they
drained swamps and built dikes and converted water
into land. And the work of the Dutch painters in the
seventeenth century was the marvel of the world. There
were also great achievements by Dutch scientists.

In the latter part of the eighteenth century, the English received a similar, though less forceful stimulus.
What had been a rather easygoing, predominantly rural
economy with only a very slowly growing population
found itself confronted, after 1750, by a comparatively
rapid growth of population, not due to any change in
family size but simply to declining mortality. The economic result was a great transformation of both agriculture and industry; not a happy period, it is true, for
those who had to live through it, but ultimately creating
the far more productive economy of the nineteenth cen-

tury. This population growth was the basic cause of extensive emigration, without which the United States would not have come into existence, to say nothing of Australia, New Zealand, and the English-speaking communities in Canada and South Africa. Without this British population growth, India too would probably not have come under the influence of European civilization. Politically, it was this century of rapid population growth that saw Britain transformed from a rigid oligarchy into a genuine democracy. Culturally, regarding the achievements of nineteenth-century England in the visual arts, probably the less said the better. But we must not forget that this was a great period in English literature, and still more so in science.

It was while this transformation was in progress, in 1798, that the Reverend Thomas Robert Malthus wrote his famous book *The Principles of Population*. Britain, with 10 million inhabitants, was, according to Malthus, already overpopulated. Though a clergyman in a country parish, he seemed quite unaware of the great improvements in agriculture that were going on during his own lifetime, still less of improvements in industrial technology.

Malthus claimed that population always grew up to the limits of subsistence. If, as sometimes happened, food supplies improved—through the settlement of new land or improved technology—population rapidly grew up to overtake them, leaving mankind in the same state of destitution as before. Population was in fact kept in check by "vice and misery," unless people adopted the "prudential restraint" he advocated, namely late marriage. He was hostile to any other form of birth limitation.

But Malthus was just wrong in his facts—alike in history, in geography, and in anthropology. So, far from being universal, rapid population growth has been a rarity in history, as we have seen. Most communities in the past have had large unused reserves of agricultural or pastoral land. In fact, Malthus's theory is almost the exact reverse of the truth. As Ester Boserup, the Danish agricultural economist, has shown, it is population growth that comes first and improvements in agricultural technology that follow, whether we look at the history of Europe, or at what is happening in present-day Africa. This takes us back to the theory that men do not adopt improvements until circumstances compel them to do so. Improving the productivity of agriculture is, for those who first undertake it, a laborious process.

Fortunately, our ancestors did not listen to Malthus. If they had, the world would be immensely different from what it is now, and a much poorer and less civilized place.

The country where Malthus did get a hearing, at any rate where his ideas were put into practice, was France. The evidence now indicates that family limitation began in France as early as 1780, nearly a century before it appeared elsewhere. Professor Sauvy, as delegate from France to the World Population Conference, posed a quite unanswerable question. If countries were right in thinking that they could make themselves richer by family limitation, he said, then France ought by now to be the richest country in the world, having practiced it for nearly two centuries. The French economic historian Marczewski, who studied the matter in great detail, blames the lack of population pressure for France's late start in industrialization in the nineteenth century.

What happened to the English in the eighteenth century happened to the Japanese in the closing decades of the nineteenth century. A population that had been kept virtually stationary for three centuries (largely, as Japanese historians ruefully record, by infanticide) began to increase in a country with extremely limited resources of agricultural land. But on their already extremely small and overcrowded farms, the Japanese succeeded in introducing great improvements in agricultural technology, raising their rice yields to four times those obtained in most Asian countries. They also industrialized with great speed and effectiveness; and by the eighteen-nineties were already successfully competing in world markets for industrial exports. Politically, Japan changed from absolute monarchy to parliamentary government, with universal suffrage introduced in 1925. After that, unfortunately, there was a reaction to military government, with consequences too well-known to all of us. The present century has not been one of cultural achievements in any way comparable with those of Japan's past. But Japan has substantial achievements in science and technology to her credit.

What happened to Britain and Japan in the eighteenth and nineteenth centuries is happening in the present century to India. The common picture of India as a country sinking ever deeper into poverty and hunger is quite mistaken. It is true that about a quarter of India's population—mostly those who made the mistake of getting born into the wrong caste—live in permanent misery and hunger. This is a disgrace to India. But it was just as much a disgrace in the past. India during the last two decades, despite some very grave errors of policy, has made far more rapid economic progress than she ever did before. I have visited India ten times, both in official and unofficial capacities, and I am getting to know something about it. Rapid population growth in India only started in the thirties. Before then, population growth had been slow—and so also had been economic progress. In 1947 I was asked to spend some time in the office of the Economic Adviser to the Indian Government. At that time, the most optimistic economists thought that it might be possible to keep production advancing ahead of population by about $\frac{1}{2}$ percent per year, though many thought that the gain in production per head might be only $\frac{1}{4}$ percent per year. They based these estimates on the records of India's own past performances. In fact, the rate of growth of production *per head* has been nearly $1\frac{1}{2}$ percent per year, or three times the most optimistic estimates of 1947. India's worst mistakes have been in agricultural policy, and food production has advanced only slightly faster than population, though its rate of growth is now rapidly accelerating. But the advances in industrial production have been striking. Though not significantly better fed, the average Indian is now better clothed, housed, medicated, and educated than his father was.

Even more striking has been the increase in savings in India. Those objecting to population growth say that bringing up children and providing for them reduces national savings. What they forget is that a country with a steadily growing population will have a high proportion of men in the most productive and saving years of their lives and a low proportion of pensioners, while a country with stationary population will be in the opposite position. And a pensioner consumes a great deal more than a child. It is in fact a demonstrated piece of economic theory (the Modigliani-Brumberg theorem) that population increase, all other things being equal, raises the rate of savings. But in India this is not only an economic theory but an observed fact. Net savings, as a percentage of net national product, which were only 5 percent in the early 1950s, in recent years have risen to 12 percent. A rise in net savings from 5 percent to 10 percent of the national product is the basic condition specified by Professor Rostow for the "takeoff."

Historians in fact will probably look back on India's takeoff in the 1950s as quite as striking as the British or Japanese takeoff in previous centuries.

It is also surely of note that during this period India has been transformed from a rigidly bureaucratic form of government, with foreign administrators in the top positions, to a parliamentary democracy with universal suffrage that—whatever its faults—is one of the very few of its kind among the developing countries.

But the reader may have in mind cases where population growth did not result in economic and political advance but led instead, as in Malthus's theory, to poverty and famine. There are indeed two such cases—Ireland in the early nineteenth century and Bangladesh in our own time. The similarities are immediately apparent. In both countries, the natural growth of industry and commerce that can be expected in a densely populated country were blocked by imperial oppression. I was commissioned to write an economic report for Pakistan in 1952. The first and strongest conclusion I drew was that if the rulers in West Pakistan did not give a fair share in the country's industrial development to the Eastern province, there would be serious trouble. This they persistently refused to do.

The conclusions we have drawn from all the countries we have examined are also true of the poorer developing countries. We are frequently told that population growth is hampering their economic development. Why hasn't anybody tried the simple exercise (see the following table) of grouping the developing countries according to their rates of population growth? The result is quite clear, and the opposite of what most people expect. The developing countries with the highest rate of population growth also have the highest rates of growth of production *per head*. There are other factors at work besides those mentioned. No businessman needs to be told that every industrial or commercial operation works more economically when it is serving a larger market. We have already seen both in theory and practice how population growth increases the rate of savings. But it also reduces per head capital requirements. Many mistaken conclusions have been drawn by applying supposed "capital-output ratios." In most industrial processes, capital requirements do not rise in full proportion to the amount we produce—indeed, in chemical engineering they have mathematical formulae showing the capital economies obtained by large-scale production. In the development of any country, there are several important "indivisibilities" such as the transport system, much of which has to be constructed, in any case, whether it is to serve a large or a small population.

Professor Hirschmann, who has made some penetrating studies of economic development, and who knows Latin America well, has pointed out that, while capital may be a scarce factor in the development of poorer countries. a still scarcer factor is indeed "enterprise," or the willingness to venture one's capital at risk in business. The rich in these countries have held their wealth too securely and too easily, and are not accustomed to business enterprise. Professor Hirschmann finds population growth in these countries economically beneficial, precisely because it does create unexpected imbalances and opportunities for windfall profits sufficient to tempt even the most sluggish investor.

Growth of Real Product per Head 1959-61 to 1966-68

Countries with population growth below 2% per year	Countries with population growth 2-2.4% per year	Countries with population growth 2.5-2.9% per year	Countries with population growth over 3% per year
Angola 1.1	Algeria −5.8	Bolivia 2.7	Brazil 1.6
Argentina 1.4	Burma 1.4	Cape Verde	Colombia 1.5
Ethiopia 2.8	Cambodia 2.0	Islands −2.6	Costa Rica 2.0
Netherlands	Ceylon 1.7	Chile 2.4	Dominican
Antilles −2.1	French-	Egypt 3.0	Republic 0.2
Portugal	speaking	Ghana 0.1	Ecuador 1.2
Guinea 0.2	Africa 1.4	Guiana 0.4	El Salvador 2.9
Uruguay −0.7	Haiti −0.7	India 0.8	Guatemala 1.8
	Indonesia −0.1	Iran 3.5	Honduras 1.7
	Jamaica 2.4	Kenya 1.6	Iraq 3.6
	Nigeria 2.7	Malawi −0.7	Israel 4.3
	Tunis 1.9	Morocco 0.8	Malaysia 3.0
		Pakistan 2.8	Mexico 3.7
		S. Korea 5.0	Nicaragua 3.9
		South	Panama 4.7
		Vietnam 2.7	Paraguay 0.8
		Sudan −0.4	Peru 2.9
		Syria 2.1	Philippines 2.0
		Tanzania 1.6	Rhodesia 0.2
		Trinidad 4.0	Surinam 2.4
		Uganda 1.5	Taiwan 6.6
			Thailand 4.4
			Venezuela 1.0
			Zambia 4.3
MEDIAN 0.6	MEDIAN 1.5	MEDIAN 1.6	MEDIAN 2.4

Source: All countries in Asia, Africa, and Latin America covered by National Accounts of Less-Developed Countries 1959-1968, OECD, Paris, 1970.

It is sometimes claimed that the extraordinary economic growth of Japan over the last twenty years is the result of population limitation. It is true that the number of children born in Japan fell very heavily after the legalization of abortion under the military government of 1949. During the '50s, the number of births was insufficient to replace the parental generation, though subsequently it has substantially increased. But during these last two decades, Japan has been drawing on her demographic capital and having it both ways. While Japanese parents had fewer young children to support, the children born in the previous decades were growing up and coming into the labor market, while Japan still had comparatively few pensioners to support. Meanwhile many married women, and also a large number of farmers were being drawn into the industrial labor force. A paradoxical result was that although Japanese families had fewer children to support, the Japanese industrialist had all the advantages of rapidly increasing population; indeed with an industrial labor force doubling in twenty years, a rate of increase found in no other country. So modern Japan is really an example of the benefits of increasing, not decreasing, the labor force. This process has now, however, come to an end, and Japanese employers are facing a serious labor shortage.

The reader may be satisfied alike with the economic, the political, the cultural effects of population growth. But still, he may say, he is concerned about the quality of life, and particularly about the lack of open space for recreation. He is quite entitled to complain. It will be these considerations, not food supply or mineral resources, that will ultimately determine the optimum population for any country, or the world.

Most of those who complain in this manner are dwellers in big cities. It is the cities that are overpopulated, not the world. There is no economic or social need in the modern world for cities to be larger than a million inhabitants, though they will have difficulty in succeeding industrially with less than half a million. How we are to transform our present industrial structure to distribute our industries and population among moderately sized towns is a matter beyond the scope of this article. It is perfectly feasible once we make up our minds to do it.

It is a virtual certainty that, during the coming century, there will be further great improvements in agricultural technology, and perhaps also in the breeding of fish. Moreover, our descendants may not want to eat as much as we do. In a century's time, even if the world's population has increased to eight times what it is now, it is probable still that less than half the world's surface will be required for agriculture and commercial forestry, and the remainder will be available for recreation, conservation, and national parks.

Pollution is not an inevitable consequence of population growth—indeed it is often seen at its worst in regions with stationary population. We could clean it up completely if we decided to do so. The worst offenders are public authorities themselves—sewage authorities who discharge their effluent untreated or half-treated, and electricity authorities filling the atmosphere with dust and sulphur dioxide. Car fumes could be checked by moderately priced attachments—we await governments that have the courage to make these attachments obligatory, as California is doing. Industrial pollution, even in the worst cases such as steel and cement, can be checked at the cost of adding about 10 percent to the capital cost of the plant. The checking of industrial effluents will be considerably cheaper. But politicians, who get most of their party funds from industrialists, will not even enforce the pollution laws they already have until public opinion becomes really compelling.

We ought to recycle all our wastes, not only to prevent pollution of the environment, but also in the long run to conserve natural resources. This applies particularly to the soil nutrients, phosphorus and potassium, which are at present lost in sewage effluent. (Our descendants could ultimately recover them from the ocean if they had to, but it would be a costly process.) The principal trouble about the treatment of sewage is its inordinate bulk. We are putting too much water down the drain, water that has been expensively pumped and filtered for us. We ought to recycle our water too, using pure water only for drinking and showers, second-class water for laundry, and third-class water for gardening, car and street washing, and lavatories.

But is it not the case, some may ask, that world population has already outrun food supplies, and that two thirds of the world are starving? This extraordinary piece of misinformation was shown by the Food Research Institute at Stanford University, an impartial and well-informed organization, to have originated when the director general of the World Food and Agriculture Organization confused two columns in a statistical table. FAO's subsequent statement that half the world was malnourished was found to be based on no evidence at all. In 1969, FAO came out with the statement that half the population of the developing countries (a very different matter from half the population of the world) were suffering from malnutrition. When I asked the director general for the evidence, he again said frankly that he had not got any.

We must not go to the other extreme, and say that hunger and malnutrition do not occur. One of the few pieces of hard evidence available, a medical survey of schoolchildren in India, showed 17 percent of them with visible signs of malnutrition. This is a very serious matter; but even so, it is far from the exaggerated figures that have hitherto been quoted. Such malnutrition in India and similar countries could be quickly put right by growing more high-protein crops such as beans and groundnuts, and by diverting to developing countries some of the large quantities of protein in fishmeal, meat-meal, and oilseed cakes, which are at present fed to animals in the advanced countries. The difficulties in the way of doing this are not agricultural or commercial, but political. While politicians in the developing countries love to talk in a general way about the world being hungry, none of them likes to get up and admit in the face of the world that his own country is suffering from malnutrition. And even when he does consent to accept help from other countries, it is very difficult to ensure that the supplies reach the children who need them and are not grafted or stolen on the way.

Professor Ehrlich states "every year food production in the developing countries falls further behind burgeoning population growth." This statement is just plain untrue. Food production in the developing countries in 1970 was 6 percent higher *per head* than it had been in 1952-1956.

Most of the developing countries have in fact done substantially better than this. Their average was brought down by a few very bad performers where food production per head substantially fell. A glance at the list shows that these were the countries that, under Russian or Chinese influence, had experimented with the collectivization of agriculture; or where agriculture had been subjected to political discrimination—Cuba, Algeria, Tunisia, Syria, Uruguay, Chile. Collectivization of agriculture in other countries, as in Russia and China, has been a recipe for creating hunger, not abundance.

But whatever conclusions can be drawn from economics, some will say, we are nevertheless consuming the world's irreplaceable resources at an intolerable rate.

"Resources" is a muddled word. Agricultural and forest products are not in any sense natural resources that are being used up. The natural resources are the climate and the soil, from which we take periodic harvests and which can be greatly enlarged if we show sufficient skill and enterprise. So far from exhausting the soil, the best modern agricultural methods progressively increase its fertility. We are only cultivating about a quarter of the world's land climatically suitable for agriculture, and in most cases, extremely badly. Without any further improvements in agricultural technology, irrigation of deserts, food from the sea, etc., but just by applying throughout the world the methods already used by good farmers in advanced countries, we could produce enough to supply American standards of consumption to ten times the world's present population.

FAO have finally decided to "blow the gaff." Dr. Pawley, their leading economist, has said frankly that their previous statements made it far too easy for people like Colin Clark to criticize. Calculating as above, but in addition making provision for the irrigation of deserts, he thinks that in the course of a hundred years the world's food production could be raised to fifty times what it is now.

There remain the minerals. But let us remind ourselves of the basic laws of chemistry. No atom of metal is ever "used up" in any human activity (except very occasionally in nuclear reactions). After we have used the metal, it still exists; it is just that its reconversion into usable form may be somewhat costly, depending on the degree to which we scatter our waste products. The basic metals, iron and aluminum, exist in the earth's crust in incredible quantities, and chemical processes are known for extracting them even from low-grade materials. The whole trouble now is that metals are far too cheap, and therefore we throw away our old cars and other waste metal, thereby disfiguring the landscape. Indeed one wishes that metals might become scarce and high-priced, thereby creating incentives to economize their use, and also to recycle all our waste products, which we ought to be doing in any case.

The only minerals that are in any sense used up are the coal and the oil that we burn. Their carbon atoms are converted to carbon dioxide in the atmosphere, and plant growth is the only way of converting it back to solid carbon. Our descendants will eventually have to stop burning coal and oil. In their place, nuclear energy will be used. The physicists think that we are not very far away from being able to replace nuclear fission by nuclear fusion, which is far more efficient, and by solar radiation converted directly to electricity. For this process, some techniques are already known.

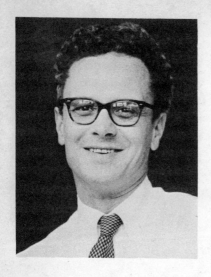

Dr. Daniel Callahan is the author of ABORTION: LAW, CHOICE, AND MORALITY *and editor of* THE AMERICAN POPULATION DEBATE.

A former staff associate at the Population Council, he is now director of the Institute of Society, Ethics, and the Life Sciences.

Daniel Callahan

LIKE MANY OTHER UNWIELDY SOCIAL ISSUES, population growth inspires contradictory attitudes: enthusiasm, apathy, hysteria, hope, fear. While there has for some time been a strong minority voice calling attention to the ills of excessive population size or growth, it has never become a leading popular cause, either in this country or anywhere else. The shouts of the few have been drowned out by the silence of the many. On the face of it, this is a curious situation. Even if there remains considerable dispute about optimal population size and growth, there is hardly any about the necessity of an eventual stabilization—zero population growth. And it requires little thought to realize that the sooner a move is made toward stabilization, the sooner it will be accomplished. Nonetheless, the message has barely gotten through, despite the large amounts of money and passion invested in trying to spread the word.

On second thought, however, it is probably not so surprising that population control has never gained a massive following or commanded the prime attention of governments. However serious the population problem, there is hardly a country in the world that cannot discover other social problems far more immediate and pressing. The Indian Government, for instance, has been fully aware of the population problem in its country for

135

over two decades; the demographic statistics can hardly
be denied. But it has been even more acutely worried
about political and military threats from China and
Pakistan, and is investing far more money in arms than
in family planning and population programs. The American black surely knows some of the costs of the excessively large family, and the price to be paid for
overcrowding. Still, the need for jobs and basic political
justice has seemed a more critical immediate need than
that of American population stabilization.

One might, of course, say about these and similar
examples that they display a possibly fatal short-sighted-
ness. If India succeeds in staving off a military invasion
in this generation, only to succumb to starvation in the
next, what is the gain? But this kind of question, for all
of its common-sense practicality, is not likely to inspire
a change in priorities. For most people, it would seem an
exercise in irrelevant abstraction to ignore present dangers in the name of possible future fatalities. Another
reason for the general apathy toward population problems relates to their very pervasiveness, which has the
effect of hiding rather than revealing them. No one dies
of overpopulation. They die as a result of malnutrition,
disease, psychological and physical pressures. One might
well *know* that the real villain is population, but this
is rarely likely to be evident to the naked eye; it takes
a demographer, an ecologist, or a nutritionist to spot
and trace the hidden relationships.

The dispelling of public apathy has not been particularly helped by the hysteria prevalent among some population-oriented groups. For one thing, the very narrow class base—white, upper middle class, highly educated—of most groups active in population work has led to suspicions about the real motivations behind the opposition to population growth. This suspicion has taken the form, at the extreme, of seeing an imperialist or genocidal plot behind a promotion of population control. More mildly, it has led to a feeling that one minority group in society is intent upon propagandizing its special values at the expense of the values of much larger, but less well-placed groups. Most importantly perhaps, the fact that some advocates of population control (Paul Ehrlich and Garrett Hardin, for instance) have raised the specter of governmental coercion has not exactly made population control look like a liberation movement.

I have stressed all these possible sources of public apathy in order to make a key point. The public at large, both in this country and elsewhere, is *never* likely to take population pressures seriously until it appears clear (a) that the price for doing so is not intolerable, and (b) that other critical social ills will not be ignored in the name of population control. Among the intolerable prices, the following can be listed: a denigration of childbearing and childrearing, state-imposed sanctions and coercions, the imposition of elite values, the minimization of present social problems in the name of solving future population problems. But is not excessive population growth itself an intolerable situation? Possibly so, for some. But it is not perceived as intolerable in the same sense or in the same way that other social problems are. Its impact, however strong, is diffuse. Its symptoms are more readily perceived than the causes, and the causes themselves are often more complex than anti-natalist propaganda admits. In this context, most of the proposed cures for population problems—with one exception, voluntary programs—appear worse than the disease.

The fact that much of the population debate in the United States has systematically confused the relationship between population growth and technological development has immensely complicated the problem of public education. The best evidence available suggests that, at most, population growth and size is an intensifier rather than the cause of air and water pollution, of the destruction of the environment, and of the spoiling of wilderness, forest, and recreation areas. Population has grown in the United States, but its rate of growth has been far outstripped by the rate of industrial and technological growth. In a word, the premise of those groups most vigorous and zealous in pressing for population control (Zero Population Growth, Inc., for instance) has been shaky and scientifically dubious. That premise was that all of the environmental and social problems of the United States could be traced to one source: too many people. That was the political plank, with Paul Ehrlich as the prophet. And it has not withstood close examination. If zero population growth was achieved immediately (a mathematical impossibility, in any case) the problems of pollution, urban crowding, ruination of parks would continue—until such time as the use of technology was brought under rational control.

The points I am making here have, for the most part, been brought forward by a relatively small group of demographers and ecologists in reaction to the early excesses of the ZPG movement. But one senses that the general public was never much captivated by those excesses in any case. Their immediate problems had to do with the war in Vietnam, inflation, unemployment rates, racism, and the like. Actually, it appears, the public has not been ready to accept either the position of ZPG or the position of those who trace the environmental problems to an uncontrolled technology. The environment has been a concern, to be sure, but as soon as stringent controls are suggested—either a control of births or a control of technology, or both together—enthusiasm quickly wanes. Clearly, both population and environment are well down on the list of the actual priorities people value. Whether they will ever be very high priorities is questionable. Nothing less than a massive change in values would suffice to bring that about, a change that would have to be accompanied by a significant reduction in the other social ills that far more bitingly capture the imagination of most people.

At root, resistance to serious change in attitudes toward procreation and technology is based on deeply

ingrained habits and values. Of the two, an unwilling-
ness to entertain the possibility of a reduction in the
scale and scope of technology may be the most stubborn
obstacle of all. There has been considerable talk of
reducing average family size. There has been practically
no talk of inducing people to give up extra automobiles;
that notion would be a cultural sacrilege of the first
order. Many millions of individuals in this country have
voluntarily limited their family size. With the exception
of fringe religious and youth groups, the number of
individuals who have voluntarily limited their consumption of the products of technology is tiny. The reason for
this is probably no great mystery. In agricultural
societies, children appear a necessity. In technological
societies, children are important, but they are not necessary for cultural or economic advancement. Moreover,
the smaller the family, the greater the chance for such
advancement. Technological progress, on the contrary,
does carry with it a perceived necessity. People can get
along without children. They cannot get along without
jobs, and jobs in our society are inextricably tied up
with the economic viability of the industrial machine.
It is not just that many people would find the sacrifice of
an extra automobile a heavy personal burden, it is also
that they are aware of the radical dislocation of the
economy that would result should the automobile industry decline in output and importance. There have
been complaints against the ZPG movement, but nothing
to compare with the violent reaction and resistance met

by those who propose the imposition of strong controls on industry in the name of pollution control or the preservation of natural resources. There has been little concern about the steadily declining birth rate, but there has been great concern about the possibility of a declining or static gross national product; the slow growth of worker productivity is already a source of alarm (2 percent per annum versus, for instance, 11 percent in Japan).

I mention these points because it is often claimed that there exist strong pro-natalist pressures in the United States. But if the real problem of population and environment is, as I have argued, far more a problem of controlling technology than population growth, then it is also necessary to recognize that the pro-natalist pressures are far less strong than the pro-technology pressures. In fact, it may be doubted that the pro-natalist pressures are very strong at all at present. The rapidly declining birth rate, which temporarily at least points to a significant shift in childbearing desires and plans, indicates that any pro-natalist pressures are relatively easy to overcome for thousands of couples (just as they were, apparently, during the Depression in the thirties).

Anti-natalist groups have tried to create the impression that it is just about impossible for Americans to remain childless or to have small families. But there has never been any solid evidence advanced that income tax deductions for dependent children, for instance, act as a positive inducement to childbearing. Nor is it clear that the kind of pressures that relatives, friends, and others put on childless couples amount to anything more than minor harassment. More significant pressures are probably brought about by discrimination against women in employment and by lingering vestiges of the view that woman's role is properly and "naturally" that of wife and mother. But the latter type of pressures are by no means unique to this country; they have existed in almost every culture in every historical era. Yet, though the struggle has not been easy, the evidence points to a sharp decline in pressure of that sort, particularly among the young, who seem quite able these days to envision having either no children or at most two. In comparative terms, the cultural and economic pressure on couples to buy an automobile is probably far stronger than to have a child; there are about $3\frac{1}{2}$ million children born each year in this country, but nearly 10 million automobiles are sold.

Nothing I have said should be taken to imply that the United States does not need a population policy or that the goal of zero population growth should not be sought as quickly as possible. Even in a time of declining birth rates, approaching zero population growth at the moment, a coherent population policy is desirable. For one thing, it has become evident that birth rates can fluctuate greatly over relatively short spans of time. No one would be surprised if there was an upturn in birth rates shortly in this country. Because of these fluctuations, the causes of which are by no means fully understood, a coherent policy might contribute to greater stability and predictability in demographic trends; that would have many advantages in addition to those that might accrue to population control. For another, there is now mounting evidence throughout the world that few, if any, nations would really find zero population growth as palatable in practice as in theory. Almost every country that has experienced low birth rates for a significant period of time—Japan, Rumania, Bulgaria, France, and Sweden, for instance—has sought to reverse the trend, well before a zero growth rate actually existed. In every case, the motivation seems to be fear of the economic consequences: a declining or an aged labor force, for example. It is no accident that all of those countries are industrialized, and that, once again, the power of a technologically based economic system can be highly potent in shaping a response to population size and growth. For the Japanese, the fear that Japan's spectacular postwar economic and industrial growth might run out of steam appears far stronger than that of overpopulation. The significance of this response is that a well-designed population policy would be one that could take account of both rises and declines in birth rates, flexible enough to go in a pro- or anti-natalist direction as the situation warrants.

I have spoken of the resistance most people would probably express toward population control programs or policies that denigrated childbearing, imposed elite values, entailed state-imposed coercion, or evaded other pressing social issues. There is a fine line between an anti-natalist population policy (which seeks only to reduce average family size to a point of demographic stabilization) and hostility toward children. At the very moment when American society is beginning to recognize the abuses and indignities children suffer, and to move toward improving their lot, other intellectual trends suggest that, for some, children are coming to be seen as the enemy, the ultimate despoilers of the private and public good life. The hostility once left toward immigrant foreigners—who also, one recalls, were accused of threatening the good life of native inhabitants—now seems capable of being transferred to children, the last immigrants, so to speak, who regularly arrive on the scene. My allusion here is only indirectly to the problem of the wanted or unwanted child. More directly I am referring to trends that would promote a culture where children as such become unwanted, quite independently of population problems or the capacity of parents to raise and care for them. I would argue that such a trend, should it develop further, will provoke considerable well-deserved hostility. It will be recognized for what it is, a basic threat not only to the children who will in fact be born and who will need care, love, and respect, but a more fundamental threat to the future, which will not exist at all without children.

Population programs that bear the stamp of minority, elite groups will provoke no less resistance. While there is no evidence to support the claim that population and family planning programs will be genocidal in intent and effect, there is more than enough to support the charge that population and family planning programs can be misused for ends having little or nothing to do with national population control. It is no secret that some look upon family planning programs as a cheap and quick way to reduce welfare rolls—far cheaper and far quicker than responding to demands for freedom and justice, urban renewal and jobs. Blacks are quick to spot the suspect motives of many who would give them only enough freedom to enable them to have smaller families, while leaving their more basic problems untouched. Beyond these considerations (which, fortunately, represent aberrations rather than the norm in family planning programs), there is the important requirement that population policies and programs represent ways of helping *all* people to achieve their most critical needs and desires. But this cannot be accomplished unless the programs and policies reflect their thinking, their values, and their participation. In matters so personal as sex and procreation, there is no reason to believe for a minute that any other method of policy formation and implementation could, as a practical political matter, succeed.

Inevitably, any serious discussion of population control must consider the full range of methods and policies that might bring about stabilization. They range the gamut from programs avowedly and actually voluntary, through those which by means of incentives or penalties would put gentle or strong pressure on people to limit family size, to those which would, if necessary, make use of such Draconian measures as enforced sterilization or abortion. As a practical matter, it is sensible to rule out the last-mentioned possibilities. It is impossible to imagine circumstances, however serious, where the public — any public — would tolerate invasions of the body for the sake of population control. Incentive and penalty schemes are more plausible, but only if designed in a way that spread their burden equally over the whole population. So far, it has been difficult to formulate plans that would, in all respects, be just and non-discriminatory. Nonetheless, such plans could undoubtedly be devised if there existed, in the first place, a sufficient sense of urgency and a consensus that purely voluntary programs have failed and will continue to fail. In this country, that point has not been reached.

It is far easier, of course, to imagine obstacles to effective population control policies than to invent viable ones. But the path of realism demands a recognition of those obstacles; too much energy has been spent on devising paper-schemes, poltically or economically unfeasible, and too little on improving present voluntary programs. Moreover, I count it a sign of moral health that the more coercive proposals get little discussion and practically no public hearing. Our society is already coercive enough, already too prone to a "law and order" mentality, to welcome further sanctions and coercions, or even to be willing to consider them. Inevitably, too, the weight of coercive policies would fall most heavily upon the poor and least educated, those whose lives are already victimized by myriad injustices.

As the above reservations indicate, the test of a population policy should encompass values far wider than a reduction of birth rates. A concern for excessive population growth has arisen not because of numbers as such; in isolation a given population size or rate of growth means nothing. The question is, What is the effect of population growth and size on human welfare? That is a question that, in order to be answered, requires some reasonably clear conception of human welfare. A threat to minimal levels of nutrition, health, and housing, traceable to population growth, would in all societies be seen as a threat to human welfare. Hence, it is easy to speak of a population problem in many poor countries and regions, particularly when these same countries also have needs that go beyond bare survival. But even in those countries, there can be tension between the values that would be enhanced by declining birth rates and other human values, also cherished, that would hinder that development. Among those values are religious convictions, family and kinship systems that place a high premium on children, protection of minority strength, and the like. Human welfare must, to have any full meaning, encompass values of that kind, whether we happen to share them or not. People do not live merely to survive; in fact, many are willing to endanger survival for the preservation of spiritual, psychological, and communal values. To speak of human welfare is implicitly to raise the question, "Whose conception of human welfare?"

If the problem of balancing cherished values is difficult enough even in countries that are desperately poor, it is hardly any easier in developed nations. What should be the motivation for population control? One answer might be the preservation or the enhancement of the "quality of life." But individuals differ notoriously about what constitutes a decent quality of life; the priorities of the poor are not necessarily the same as those of the affluent, nor do urban dwellers necessarily want the same things as those living in rural or suburban areas. All might agree that a basic minimal standard of food, clothing, and housing is essential. Beyond that, however, there is little agreement on just how much technology individuals need to sustain a fulfilled life. I do not doubt that it is possible to develop a consensus of a general sort on problems of this kind. But, even if developed, the chances are good that it will represent more the views of the majority than of the minority. And that would still leave open the delicate question of the extent to which the majority could impose its views on others in the name of population control.

Both constitutionally and ethically, it is doubtful that coercive sanctions could be introduced for the sake of a certain quality of life. Only a very direct threat to survival would provide the necessary grounds; and there is no evidence now that survival is at stake in the United

States. Human beings require liberty, particularly in a matter as personal as that of procreation. They also require just treatment and a recognition that justice presupposes equality under law and, at times, variable treatment in order that past injustices may be corrected. The goal of a population policy cannot, in the end, be simply that of reducing population growth or effecting a better population distribution. The goal of a population policy is human welfare, physical, psychological, and ethical. The test of any policy will be whether it contributes to that goal.

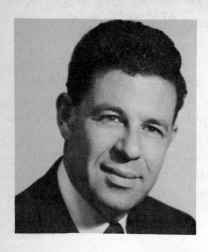

Chairman of the Department of Sociology at Columbia University, Dr. Etzioni has also served as consultant to our Government's Public Health Service, Office of Economic Opportunity, and Committee on the Causes and Prevention of Violence.

In 1968, he won a Guggenheim Fellowship, and in 1967, the William Mosher Award.

He is on the editorial board of the INTERNATIONAL JOURNAL OF GROUP TENSIONS. *His book,* MODERN ORGANIZATIONS, *has been translated into ten languages. His other works include* STUDIES IN SOCIAL CHANGE, COMPLEX ORGANIZATIONS: A SOCIOLOGICAL READER, READINGS ON MODERN ORGANIZATIONS, *and with his wife Eva as co-author,* SOCIAL CHANGE: SOURCES, PATTERNS, AND CONSEQUENCES. *Dr. Etzioni also has to his credit an impressive number of professional books and articles.*

Amitai Etzioni

THE DEBATE ABOUT POPULATION CONTROL—should we have it and what kind we should have—is in large part a false issue. There is now no such thing and very likely there can be no such thing as population *control*. Control implies to be in charge, to guide, to direct. For instance, I can control the temperature of a room to a single degree by setting the thermostat, or control the direction of my car to the very spot it comes to stop. But no person, corporation, or government can set the rate of population growth at zero or 2.3 percent or 1.6 percent or any other precise point.

Control assumes both a capacity to understand the present situation and, at very least, a basic understanding of the levers that could change the condition. In the United States we have rough measures of present population size and growth rate. (The picture in other nations is often much foggier.) But in order to control we need to know more than that; we also have to know where we are headed, at least in the near future. This we cannot do yet. There are, of course, numerous predictions, projections, forecasts; but they are often significantly off the mark.

Two incidents involving the 1970 census give an indication of the range of error and of the difficulties involved in a task even as relatively simple as counting. Before the census tally, estimates of age distribution in

the population included half of the population in a
bracket of twenty-five years or under. But the census
uncovered a median-age of 27.9, a difference of almost
three full years, from what the experts had generally
believed.[1] In New York City, counting the number of
residents turned out to be a major problem. In August,
1970, a preliminary census report showed New York
City's population down 750,000 from 1960 although the
Census Bureau did admit that there might be as many
as 210,000 people who had not been counted, a category
they named "missing." John C. Cullinane, Regional Census Director, was quoted as saying that, in light of urban
population trends, a drop of one-half million "should
not be surprising." But the fun was just beginning. On
September 9 the Census Bureau issued a new report that
gave the city a drop of only 10,254. Three days later the
bureau indicated it may have missed 70,000 people who
were away in April, and in November gave a revised
"final" count that showed the city's population *up* 16,773
from 1960. However, the "final" count was not quite
final. In May, 1971, almost a full year after the census
returns were in, the Census Bureau discovered that it
had "lost" 28,000 New York City residents in its computer![2]

When the task is prediction, rather than just count-

---

[1] *New York Times*, Jan. 17, 1972.

[2] For accounts of the changes in Census Bureau reports see the *New
York Times* of August 22, September 5, November 16, 1970, and
May 23, 1971.

ing, the magnitude of mistakes may be enormous. For instance, among the slightly less than 7 million poor and near-poor women between the ages of fifteen and forty-four, there were more than 1 million fewer births in the period 1966-1970 than had been expected on the basis of 1960-1965 fertility rates.[3]

How can we control anything if we don't know where it's going? It's like driving in the dark, with very dim lights. But imagine the difficulties if, on top of the darkness, the car had faulty standard gears and the driver had only used automatic. While a full comprehension of controlling factors is not necessary, no process can be guided without a minimum of practical knowledge; thus, our imaginary driver doesn't need a degree in engineering but he does need to know which way the car will move when he switches gears.

Consider the situation in regard to population. Some *believe* that wide distribution of contraceptives will reduce the population growth while others hold that it will only make people shift from one method of birth control to another. Some believe that population growth is an autonomous process while others suggest it is all a matter of basic social changes.[4] The reasons these opinions can roam so freely and intensely is that we know so little, and that what we believe we know is often insuffi-

[3] *New York Times*, March 2, 1972.

[4] For a comprehensive review of various measures and their ethical and political acceptability as well as their efficiency, see Bernard Berelson, *Studies in Family Planning*, No. 38 (February, 1969).

ciently documented. There are no debates about how to set a thermostat.

More importantly, no government commands either the power or the consensus population *control* requires. Here and there population-control advocates let their fancy run free. They see a government sneaking a contraceptive drug into the milk (liquor would be better) or issuing a birth quota. However, a government that resorts to such means is not likely to last long; governments are regularly overthrown for far less cause then preventing people from having children. And if a birth quota were somehow established, people would surely "bootleg" children at least as freely as they bootlegged booze when it was prohibited.

The fact of the matter is that most people seem not to subscribe to the alarmist views about (a) the future pace of population growth; (b) the dire consequences of such growth; or (c) the desirability of having other things rather than children. Most people do not believe that we are moving toward a day in which there will only be standing room in this globe. Thus, a 1971 Gallup poll found that only 41 percent of those polled thought that population growth was a major issue requiring immediate action. While 81 percent thought population growth might sometimes affect their quality of life, only 54 percent showed concern about the possibility.[5] It should also be realized that the poll did not ask the respondents to weigh this concern against a desire for children. And

[5] *New York Times,* April 16, 1971.

in addition, people seem to feel that if the government decided to do so, it could feed and clothe 4 billion people, even if it meant cutting back in space tours and arms races.

Last, in the most telling of all ballots, in their real-life decisions, many "voters" opt for more children and fewer "things" as a "better" way of life. When a child is conceived, parents may well be unaware of what he or she will cost themselves or the society. Actually, at this stage, they may not think at all. But most, looking back at their decision, seem quite unwilling, at least for now, to legislate or tolerate population control. Nor can they, for reasons I cannot explore here, be "sold" on such a policy by government or foundation propaganda.[6]

If we are not controlling population growth (which is quite obvious) and cannot do so at least in the foreseeable future, what can we do? As in many other policy areas, we are really *spot interveners*. We launch a health program here (which reduces infant mortality); we set up abortion clinics there; we have a program of vasectomies, etc. Like a frantic visitor to Paris charging up the steps of the Eiffel Tower and down the halls of the Louvre, we do a little of everything and not much of anything. Americans openly advocate "pluralistic" approaches, minimal government role, and are skeptical

[6] For discussion of this point as well as additional theoretical background, on the concept of controlling social processes and the elements needed to bring about such control, see Amitai Etzioni, *The Active Society* (New York: Free Press, 1968).

about master planning, grand theories, and overall reviews. Other nations may put a more rationalistic gloss over the same activities. They launch grand drives to provide every woman in the fertile age with an IUD, show every teen-ager a film about birth control or whatnot. These drives are quite large in the millions of items, dollars, or people involved—compared to the American efforts (if you take those of any one source). But as a rule, they are far from considerable in terms of the progress they effect, the control achieved. In fact, their effect on population control is usually so small and hidden, it is hard to measure! All in all, planning is more effective if the problem is approached in terms of opportune targets and spot intervention rather than saturation programs. Thus, if a social-studies text is prepared, the ministry of education (this is the way it is done in many countries) may include a chapter on the techniques of birth control. Or if young males are being drafted, one may explain to them the facts of life, as part of their basic training.

Before I suggest where some of the best targets seem to be, let me indicate some of the fairer and more obvious criteria for their selection. A negative criterion has already been established: We do not require that these targets fit into a master plan, although their side effects on other efforts surely deserve a hearing. Secondly, of course, relative cost effectiveness must be taken into account somehow, preferably with a big grain of salt—i.e., loosely—rather than trying to get hard, detailed figures. That is, approaches that deal with small numbers—each requiring an expensive treatment with low probability of success—must be avoided in favor of those that deal with large numbers, are inexpensive (in money *and* in the kind of manpower they use), and have a high probability of a payoff. Also, such programs should require as few steps and as little coordination as possible, and otherwise be relatively free from the possibility of bureaucratic tampering.

While few would question the cost-effective criteria in abstract, in practice they are often ignored. Thus, most nations engaged in birth control spend millions on what sociologists call formal communications—three-colored posters, ads, billboards. Evidence that these methods pay off in changing attitudes toward family size (or any other deep-seated attitude) is rather slim.

More generally there is reason to believe that educational efforts, in the broadset sense of the term, are among the least cost-effective. A report by Elizabeth Drew demonstrates that it costs $88,000 to save a life via driver education as compared to $87 if seat belts are provided.[7] Similarly, methadone is vastly more cost-effective than attempts at education or psychological rehabilitation of drug addicts.

In the birth-control area, rather than trying to change preferences of people, it seems more effective to focus first on those millions of unwanted pregnancies,

[7] Elizabeth Drew, "HEW Grapples with PPBS," *The Public Interest*, No. 8, Summer, 1967, p. 16.

i.e., where to one extent or another, the preference exists and the willingness to do something about it is often present. I do not know, I believe no one can really tell, if just dealing with the unwanted pregnancy will or will not solve the problem. Obviously the answer will differ not only from country to country, but over time as well. Quite possibly, by the time most of those who now want assistance, but do not know where to find it or know how to use it, will be helped, another population with different characteristics and desires will have become the appropriate target. In any event, for reasons of both costs and ethics, it makes little sense to try to change preferences if those who already have a preference have not been served.

And, it is clear that the number of unwanted pregnancies, even in the U.S.A., is very considerable. In a survey of 5,600 American women of childbearing age, Charles Westoff found that 26 percent of the children born were due to unwanted conceptions. (If unmarried women had been included in the sample, the effect would have been to push the rate still higher.) In a secondary analysis of his data, he found that unwanted fertility accounts for between 35 and 45 percent of the population growth in this country.[8] Another source estimates that about 15 percent of all American babies born between 1966 and 1970, some 2,650,000, were unwanted:

[8] L. Bumpass and C. F. Westoff, "The 'Perfect Contraceptive' Population," *Science*, Vol. 169, No. 3951, September 18, 1970, p. 1178. Secondary analysis reported in *New York Times*, October 29, 1969.

> *Had these children not been conceived,
> the fertility rate of the average American
> woman would have been 2.7 children for
> those years, instead of the actual rate of
> 3.0 children. To achieve zero population
> growth, where births approximately cancel
> out deaths, women would have to bear an
> average 2.1 children.*[9]

How to help those with existing preferences? Surprisingly often, all they seem to need are the means and the know-how. Thus, two reasons so many unmarried youngsters get pregnant against their will are that contraceptives are not readily available and that the knowledge of how to use them is still not nearly as widely spread as one would assume in the age of sexual revolution. For example, while in Sweden one can buy condoms from vending machines day and night, this is not the case in most of the U.S.A. nor in most other countries. A study of the problems involved in delegating the dispensation of birth-control pills from MD's to pharmacists, or even to supermarkets (complete with warnings for those who have diabetes or similar medical histories), may suggest that this might be preferable to existing arrangements. Also basic information about birth control must still be disseminated even in modern societies like ours.

I realize that the notion of a preference is not sim-

[9] *Newsweek*, March 27, 1972.

ple. Some women favor birth control, but not when they consciously or subconsciously wish to marry the man with whom they have intercourse. Some men favor birth control, but not if it involves fidgeting after reaching a state of arousal.

Generally, preference is to be treated as a continuum rather than a dichotomy. That is, people are not for or against birth control: They have varying degrees of acceptance or rejection. This suggests that we not seek to focus on those who simply want birth control, but first of all on those who want it most; then—next most, and so on. A study would be necessary to establish exactly which groups these are. But we do have some rough, preliminary suggestions. For instance, Bumpass and Westoff found that the likelihood of a child's being wanted is lower when income or education of the parents is lower, and when there are already children. While only 15 percent of the children born to parents with incomes over $10,000 are unwanted, 34 percent of those born to parents with incomes under $3,000 are unwanted. Among mothers with less than a high-school education, 26 percent of their children are unwanted, compared to 13 percent among those who went to college.

Even more striking are the figures for birth order. Only 4 percent of first children and 6 percent of second children are unwanted. But among the third and fourth children, 18 percent and 25 percent are unwanted, 39 percent of the fifth, and 45 percent of the sixth or later. Among blacks fully 72 percent of the sixth or later children are not wanted by at least one parent.[10]

Another relevant consideration is most easily made by relating an incident that occurred during one of the few times I became involved in high-level policy making on this matter. A small group of consultants was called in by the president of one of the major foundations engaged in population programs in several countries. In those days, the IUD was a great and promising novelty and we spent the first hour of our consulting day listening to its promise. We were then told not to worry about the technologies (this, we were told, would be taken care of by another division), but to focus on motivation, attitudes, values; how could these be modified to be more favorable to birth control? But it soon became evident that one cannot separate these two considerations; different birth-control techniques simply assume different levels and kinds of motivation. Given, say, weak acceptance, some techniques will do much better than others. Thus, coitus interruptus seems to require more "will power" than taking a pill; taking a pill regularly requires more modern or bureaucratic behavior than using a condom; and the IUD, which can be inserted once and then forgotten, requires less motivation and more opportunities for settling conflicting feelings than the other methods.

Unfortunately, the last years have shown that IUD is far from a simple, safe, and reliable method. Accord-

[10] Bumpass and Westoff, p. 1181.

ing to Dr. F. S. Jaffe of Planned Parenthood-World Population, it has a failure rate of 7 percent over a 12-month span. The comparable figure for pills is 4 percent.[11] Moreover, in a study of seven thousand IUD users in Taiwan, L. P. Chow found that 7 percent of the women were pregnant and 11 percent had accidentally expelled the device within a year. After three years, 14 percent of the users were pregnant, 36 percent had had the device removed, and 15 percent had expelled it. So, far from being permanent, the IUD was still active and effective in only about one third of the women after three years.[12]

Thus, despite all the investment and effort, there is still no simple, inexpensive, reliable, safe birth-control means that can be used without medical or paramedical assistance, and that once taken need not be retaken until it is deliberately removed or canceled by an antidote. *That is, there is no means of birth control for the weakly motivated.* This would seem to imply that once we have provided service to the highly motivated first, the need for new technologies will become particularly acute. Since it takes years to develop one, it seems to me that further research and development in this area is urgently

[11] F. S. Jaffe, "Toward Reduction of Unwanted Pregnancy," *Science*, Vol. 174, No. 4005, October 8, 1971, p. 120.

[12] L. P. Chow, "A Study of the Demographic Impact of an IUD Programme," *Population Studies*, Vol. 22, No. 3, November, 1968, p. 355.

needed, despite the widely held notion that the problem is not technical.

Quite deliberately, I left to the end two caveats. First, there is much more to population control than birth control. In effect, death control and health services are equally significant. But the points made above in reference to birth control apply to them as well.

Second, a major school of thought has recently stressed that we should focus on societal change, specifically, on urbanization, rather than on the narrower aspects of population control. It is pointed out that these matters are integral facts of a larger societal dynamics and cannot be viewed independently of it: The best way to treat the details is to view them as part of a larger process. For instance, as societies modernize, people live longer and have fewer children.[13] This approach seems to me to be intellectually valid; indeed without it we would see leaves, not trees—let alone the forest. However, when it comes to policy making, we must focus on those matters that have "play" and can be effected by the resources we can put to use. Surely no one expects that urbanization will reduce the birth rate, or that nothing of significance can be achieved about the population level unless we urbanize further.

[13] For an example of this argument, see Kingsley Davis, "Population Policy: Will Current Programs Succeed?" *Science*, Vol. 158, November 19, 1967, pp. 130-39.

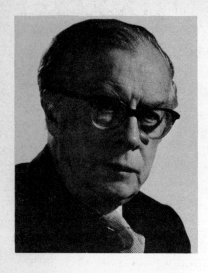

Sir Julian Sorell Huxley, British biologist and author, is well-known to the concerned American citizen as a former Director General of UNESCO and president of the Eugenics Society, and as a Galton, William Alanson White, and Sloan-Kettering lecturer.

Sir Julian, who was knighted in 1958, has been awarded both the Darwin and Darwin-Wallace Commemorative medals.

He is the author and editor of over forty important books, among them THE SCIENCE OF LIFE *(with H. G. and G. P. Wells),* THE HUMAN CRISIS, SCIENTIFIC RESEARCH AND SOCIAL NEEDS, EVOLUTION, THE MODERN SYNTHESIS, EVOLUTION AND ETHICS, *and* ESSAYS OF A HUMANIST.

Julian Huxley

I HAVE BEEN INTERESTED IN THE PROBLEM of population growth and its effects for nearly half a century, and I have supported family planning associations and clinics from the time they were first set up. I prefer now to think mainly in terms of population control, instead of merely controlling the size of separate families. Of course, it is important to remember the misery caused to mothers by excessive childbearing, to fathers who have to earn enough to support a large family, and to the unwanted child, often growing up without sufficient care and love; but these problems are only part of the greater one of excessive population.

In any case, if I am asked whether a country's and the world's population should be regulated, my answer is *Yes*; and if the question is whether world population should be stabilized—if possible, somewhat below its present level—my answer is again *Yes*.

There has been much opposition to the idea of family limitation, and still more to that of limiting whole populations. I remember with wry humor what happened over forty years ago when I gave a talk on the radio on "the population problem." At the time, I emphasized the fact that continued population growth—which is inevitably growth at compound interest; "exponential" is the jargon phrase— is bound eventually to involve disaster. I anticipated overcrowding, damage to the environment, pollution, a lower quality of human living, and in the long run (indeed, not very long) starvation and misery. Accordingly, I ended by pressing for better facilities for obtaining advice on birth control.

As a result, I was summoned to the presence of the then director of the British Broadcasting Corporation, the formidable bushy-eyebrowed Scotsman, Sir John Reith (later Lord Reith). I was put on the mat like any errant schoolboy, and told that I had "polluted the ether" —or did Sir John say "my" ether?—with such a disgusting suggestion.

Reith, that Wuthering Heights of a man, as Sir Winston Churchill once called him, is now dead; and resistance to the idea of family planning (and even of general population control) has strikingly declined—at least in Western Europe and the U.S.A. It has declined in direct proportion to our added knowledge about the general ecology of our planet, and man's effect upon it.

When we view world population in historical perspective, its growth becomes really frightening. The total number of human beings, it seems, cannot have reached 20 (or at most 25) million by perhaps 6,000 B.C., after which rudimentary agriculture permitted a fairly rapid increase. Yet man as a species had already been in existence for well over a million—some say for 2 million—years.

The start of civilization and organized trade boosted

multiplication again, so that the most probable figure for world population was around 100 million by 1,000 B.C., when the discovery of iron smelting must have given it a further boost. Yet it cannot have reached 250 million (a quarter of an American billion) till well after the birth of Christ, probably in the third century A.D. From then on, we have only estimated figures, but migration and improved agricultural methods must have steadily increased man's numbers, with occasional setbacks due to wars, famines, and plagues.

The first moderately accurate estimates are those for the middle of the seventeenth century, when total population numbered about 500 million, and the percentage of its annual rate of increase probably about 0.5. Since then—with the rise of technology, improvements in medicine, the spread of knowledge and better agricultural methods—both its absolute size and rate of increase have risen steadily. Thus, the annual rate of world increase reached 1 percent well within the present century, and is now already over 2 percent.

Let us remember that an annual increase of 2 percent means doubling the population in about thirty-five years, and that one of 3 percent will double it in twenty-five years. Even the modest 1 percent increase rate toward which Britain (and other industrially advanced countries) is tending will double our numbers in seventy years, which is a single Biblical lifetime. A reduction of the world population increase rate to $1\frac{1}{2}$ percent would still double our numbers in under fifty years, less than civilized man's average life span. This means that the present world total of about 3 billion will reach at least 6 billion by the end of the century, when many of our grandchildren will still be alive. Indeed, the total may well be higher, since modern medicine is enabling an increasing proportion of children to grow up and produce children in their turn.

The effect of this shows itself especially in so-called underdeveloped countries. Thus, in India life expectation was under twenty years at the dawn of this century; it increased to thirty-two by 1940, and is still going up.

The reduction of infant mortality by the availability of better health services operates in the same way, but even more spectacularly. In 1900, in various so-called developing communities (e.g. East African tribes), mortality in the first year of life took from a third to half the babies. Even in advanced or developed countries, similar drops have occurred. To take but one example: in 1900, the rate of infant mortality in Britain was over 15 percent; today, the percentage is down to 2 percent.

I remember reading of one particularly striking case of improved medical care leading to an explosive increase of total population. D.D.T. virtually wiped out malaria in Ceylon in seven years, and the death rate was almost halved. The birth rate did not drop, but probably increased slightly. In any case, the rate of annual increase went up to a point at which doubling the population will take only thirty years. How can any nation cope with such rapid change—even with aid from more fortunate countries, or from the United States?

With this appalling prospect of a world crowded with at least 14 billion people within eighty years, no wonder that U Thant, in his last year of office as Secretary General of the U.N., said in an official speech: "Members of the United Nations have perhaps ten years left to launch a global partnership, to curb the arms race, to improve the human environment [I myself would have said "to prevent further deterioration of the environment"], to defuse the population explosion, and to supply the required momentum for further development"—including, of course, not only economic development, but also cultural progress.

He went on to say that if such a partnership were not forged, and operative within the next decade, man's problems will have reached such staggering proportions that they will be beyond our capacity to control.

Alarming words, but U Thant is no alarmist. He was merely drawing rational conclusions from known facts and present trends; and in my view, the most threatening trend he mentioned is that toward increase of population.

"Be fruitful and multiply" is all too easy a command. It was necessary at the time it was made and for centuries before, while disease was cutting man down. It is so no longer, with our better conditions and more efficient medical achievements.

The frightening fact about population growth— which is always at some rate of compound interest—is its apparent inevitability, its juggernautlike capac ty to crush the quality of human life, despite setbacks to its advance. Thus the Black Death killed off nearly half the population of western Europe in a few decades after its introduction from the East in 1348. Yet, by 1400 the population had recovered to what it had been before the plague first erupted, and its compound-interest progress continued as if there had been no plague at all.

Similarly, I shall never forget the graph Professor Raymond Pearl showed me of European and North American population in the first sixty years of the present century. Despite immense losses caused by two world wars (and by the influenza epidemic that followed the first world war)—losses which amounted to well over 20 million—Pearl's graph merely showed a sharp downward nick and by 1950 was back again on its accelerating course, toward the 14 billion expected by 2050.

Some form of population control has been practiced by all human societies; many primitive people exposed unwanted babies, especially girl babies, as did such highly civilized people as the classical Greeks. Many tribes limit their families by traditional herbal agencies, or by modifying sexual intercourse so as to make it infertile. By historic times, more elaborate contraceptive methods were practiced. Egyptian princesses used an I.U.D. (intrauterine device) consisting of a plug made of sacred crocodile dung mixed with honey, and later flushed out with a sort of syringe. Women of classical Rome certainly knew most of the tricks needed to prevent conception, as did women in medieval Europe. In the eighteenth century, thanks to that genius Colonel Cundum (whose name, slightly altered, is immortalized in the condom he invented), mechanical devices for men came into general use. And now chemistry has come to our aid with The Pill, crowning years of careful research, while abortion and sterilization are legally accepted in a few countries, such as Britain, Sweden, and some North American states.

I must now point out some of the present difficulties caused by differences in population growth (and size) in different countries.

Japan, though its rate of population increase is low—just over 1 percent, about the same as that of the U.S.A.—is grossly overcrowded, with a population of about 112 million and an annual increase of well over a million. When the country was defeated in World War II, large numbers of Japanese settled in other territories were forced to return to their homeland; to counter this major influx of population, an intensive birth-control campaign was instituted, in which abortion as well as sterilization and conventional contraceptive methods were advocated. This brought the birth rate down, but only to where the increase was still over 1 percent per annum. The situation is still critical, and in desperation, a new militant movement has arisen. For the moment it is only a background threat, but further crowding could well force desperate attempts to conquer more living space.

China, the most populous country in the world, totals over 700 million, with an annual increase of over 14 million.

The total population of Australia is less than 13 million, and new settlement is difficult because of the desertic nature of its interior. No wonder they refuse almost all Asian immigrants. It is quite unfair to accuse them of racist prejudice; they naturally want to prevent overpopulation of their continent. After all, it is their country!

India today contains nearly 700 million people, and its annual increase is higher than China's, $2\frac{1}{2}$ percent as against a little over $1\frac{1}{2}$ percent. In both countries, the plight of the people is aggravated by deforestation, but India, with its dusty plains, is the most unfortunate of the two. Matters are so grave that, besides reducing the land to desert, many of its half-million villages lack fuel, and have to make do with dry cowpats instead. Of these there are plenty for India's cows are sacred; indeed, these scraggy sacred cows are now so numerous and eat so much of what might otherwise feed people that birth control for cows is now being seriously considered, and a special line of contraceptive devices is being manufactured. A birth-control campaign for humans is also being pushed; indeed, birth control for men (by vasectomy) is being rewarded, in some states by money payment or by the gift of a transistor radio— fewer people but more noise! Yet, ignorance and apathy are holding up the general campaign. Here also, as else-

where, prejudice is at work; underprivileged minorities—
the blacks in the U.S. and many Africans in Africa—
believe that birth control is advocated by the powers
that be to kill off the despised minorities.

Haiti, already grossly overpopulated, is still increasing by nearly 2 percent a year. Jamaica is so overcrowded that tens of thousands of its blacks emigrate to
the U.S. or Britain every year. Mexico is growing at a
rate of about $2\frac{1}{2}$ percent per annum; and Brazil by about
2 percent, which means that the settled regions are getting overcrowded, and large numbers of surplus people
are penetrating ever farther into the interior, taking land
from the native Indians, killing them if they resist,
infecting them with fatal diseases, and driving them
into the alien jungle.

Perhaps the highest increase in the world is in Latin
America, where a high rate of immigration is reinforced
by a high birth rate, owing to the official Roman Catholic
ban on "unnatural" birth-control methods. These include
all man-made contraception devices, leaving only the
so-called "rhythm" method of mating only during the
few days of the woman's monthly cycle when she lacks
an ovum to be fertilized. Unfortunately the cycle is not
accurately fixed in nature, and also it is difficult for
women, especially uneducated women, to remember
just when their infertile period occurs. Attempts to
overcome these difficulties were made when UNESCO,
together with the W.H.O. and F.A.O., set up a few birth-
control clinics in India; the women were provided with

necklaces of thirty beads, some specially colored to indicate "no-baby days," the safe period, the rest with a different color, denoting "baby days"; but the women got muddled and failed to use the necklaces properly (or, more probably, human nature intervened).

The situation is perhaps worse in Roman Catholic countries; but even so, many couples defy their Church's ban and practice birth control. Unfortunately, this does not apply to the more religious (or more superstitious), and because most Latin-American peoples are very religious and unwilling to incur the reproof of their priests, birth rates here are among the highest in the world.

Luckily, the more intelligent Catholics, both lay and clerical, are beginning to realize the personal and social misery caused by the ban; and I believe that, within a generation, Catholic countries will practice birth control. Remembering U Thant's doomful words, however, we must ask whether this will not be too late.

Clearly, the time is past when augmenting a nation's military and political power was of prime importance, and was measured by the size of its population. Mechanization and the invention of weapons of mass destruction have made quantity of men less important, while conciliation and arbitration of international disputes have become more frequent.

Today, we think more of status; and a nation's status is now increasingly measured by the quality of life it makes available by its amenities and interests, by the standard of living it provides for its people. Such aims cannot be achieved if the population is allowed to grow beyond control, either excessively or haphazardly. We must face the fact that this is happening today.

The disastrous evils following the explosion of man—this cancer of the planet—are all too evident to need further stressing. Climatic and ecological disturbances, pollution, extinction of many animals and plants, over exploitation of natural resources, unbearable living conditions in overcrowded cities leading to sickness of body and soul—the list is endless and horrifying.

The upshot is clear. We need to wake up from the strange euphoria of the past, when no thought was given to the limits of Earth's resources and their endurance; when the password for any and every activity of man was *Expand*. We are now seeing the results of this misguided, indeed insane attitude, and find ourselves on the brink of disaster.

What then can we do to save the world—and ourselves? There is not much time before the point of no return.

I agree entirely with U Thant that what he calls a global partnership is needed, a global partnership pressing for and demanding global action. My suggestion would be that the United Nations set up a special body to deal with the problem: a *U.N. Agency for Population*. This would insist on each member state setting up its own population-control commission, including at least one representative of the U.N. as adviser; it would proclaim a Population Decade (as the U.N. has done for conservation).

Public opinion is already alerted, though perhaps confusedly. A special publicity campaign should be set up to inform the public further, to put the evidence before its conscience. Politicians, who hitherto have been more anxious to maintain their popularity than to face the facts, should be urged to direct their minds and energies to this all-important problem. Family allowances should be reversed, diminishing financial benefits for every child after the second, instead of increasing them as the family grows.

I am sure that most tensions in the world would be reduced once the pressure of population was lessened. If once we manage to conquer this gravest danger of all, this senseless overproduction of men, we shall be able to conquer other dangers.

Having coped with the population monster, could we not then pay attention to the most fundamental of all questions: *What are people for?*

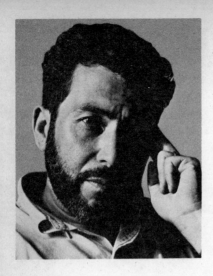

Nat Hentoff, a staff writer for THE NEW YORKER *and a columnist for* THE VILLAGE VOICE, *is an Associate Professor at New York University's Graduate School of Education.*

A member of the Board of Directors of the New York Civil Liberties Union, Mr. Hentoff is also a member of the Free Speech Association Committee of the American Civil Liberties Union. He writes regularly for the ACLU's CIVIL LIBERTIES *journal and also contributes—on a wide range of subjects—to* COMMONWEAL, THE NEW YORK TIMES, *and other publications.*

Author of many books, Nat Hentoff is best known for OUR CHILDREN ARE DYING, JAZZ COUNTRY, *and* THE NEW EQUALITY. *He lectures frequently at colleges and universities throughout the United States, and is a 1972-73 Guggenheim Fellow, concentrating on "the nature and process of learning to be a free citizen."*

Nat Hentoff

I AM FOR POPULATION CONTROL, but I am against compulsory population control.

My credo applies equally to every woman's right to an abortion on demand, to every man's right to a vasectomy, and to the right of every man and woman to reproduce.

It is a position that presents problems if one agrees in large part with the new Malthusianism. And I do.

However, unlike B. F. Skinner, I not only believe in free will but I also believe that a sufficiently informed citizenry will voluntarily choose to limit the number of its progeny.

I may be wrong. I can well foresee a governmental attempt at compulsory population control within a generation. If that happens, a vital element of constitutional democracy will have been destroyed.

As the U. S. Supreme Court declared in 1891 (*Union Pac. Ry. v. Botsford*):

> *No right is held more sacred, [n]or is more carefully guarded . . . than the right of every individual to the possession and control of his own person, free from all restraint or interference by others unless by clear and unquestionable authority of law.*

179

As was well said by Judge Cooley:

> *The right to one's person may be said to be a right of complete immunity: to be let alone.*

In view of subsequent Supreme Court decisions climaxed in 1965 by *Griswold v. Connecticut*—which maintained the individual's constitutional right to decide whether and when to have a child—it is inescapable that any law that prevents or mandates birth control is unconstitutional.

The constitutional and free-will arguments aside, I agree entirely with American Civil Liberties Union attorney Harriet Pilpel that it is far too soon to seriously discuss compulsory measures while so many obstacles remain to voluntary birth control.[1]

Of immediate priority, for example, is the striking down of all state laws that interfere with abortion. Furthermore, greatly increased research funds are needed to find more effective contraceptives; and as Ms. Pilpel emphasizes:

> *Little is done to assure the delivery of the contraceptives we now could have available to all; it is estimated that even in the United States, something like four and one-half million low-income women are without effective access to contraceptives.*

[1] *Civil Liberties,* November, 1971.

She makes the corollary point that various studies indicate *"desired* family size among the poor and indigent is smaller than the size preferred by the upper and middle income groups." [Emphasis added.] In this, as in so many other areas, freedom of choice is restricted by one's place in the hierarchical class order. The higher one's place, the more able one is to implement desire.

Nor, it should be noted, is voluntary sterilization easily available to those who want it, although the procedure is presently legal in all but one state. The barriers in this regard are those set up by doctors and, hospital administrators—and not only Catholic doctors and Catholic hospital administrators. Such arbiters act, too, to restrict the individual's freedom of choice on what he or she chooses to do with his or her body.

We will not know the effectiveness of voluntary population control, therefore, until *all* these present limitations on the freedom *not* to have children are removed. Accordingly, the role of the state should be, as Ms. Pilpel underlines, to act—

> *to make real freedom of choice possible. It should do everything from repealing repressive laws, to encouraging research in contraceptive and abortifacient technology, to ensuring effective delivery of services on a voluntary basis to all segments of our population, to waging educational campaigns.*

It seems to me that those who would work to impose compulsory population control without waiting to see the results of full voluntary control have an elitist view of the intelligence of the masses. Once again, certain "experts" are claiming to know what the people ought to be forced to do for their own good without really undertaking to find out how "backward" the people actually are.

The U. S. Census Bureau reported on February 16, 1972, that "the number of children that American women expected to bear dropped so sharply between 1967 and 1971 . . . that the nation is fast approaching zero population growth rates among younger women." One of the reasons, as I can attest from many conversations with young people throughout the country in recent years, is that the message concerning the ecological results of an unchecked birth rate is decidedly getting through.

Also worth considering with regard to the potential of voluntarism is the Planned Parenthood-World Population study that disclosed that:

> Birth rates among lower-income women declined so sharply in the late nineteen-sixties that they bore a million fewer children than they would have at the earlier rates . . . In absolute terms, the study showed a significant narrowing of the historic divergence between the fertility rate of poorer, and richer women . . . The

*change was even steeper among poor black
women.* [2]

Again, this development is taking place during a
time of scarcity of information and research concerning
birth-control methods. Consider, then, the much larger
potential of fully informed voluntarism.

The facilitation of voluntary birth control would
also avoid an otherwise serious political problem if any
compulsory action were attempted. Many black people—
and members of other minority groups—fiercely oppose
compulsory birth control as another white way of
achieving "genocide" (to use a frequent term in black
denunciations of compulsory population limitation).
However, blacks and other minority groups are not opposed to voluntarism. In December, 1971, a Nashville
conference of black physicians, dentists, medical and
dental students, health workers, politicians, and consumers utterly rejected compulsory population control
but simultaneously declared that family planning is
acceptable "if it is an integral part of a comprehensive,
total health service."

Similarly, on April 9, 1972, the steering committee
of the National Association of Black Social Workers,
meeting in Nashville, announced that:

> *its position on family planning would be
> to oppose forced or coerced birth control*

[2] *New York Times,* March 3, 1972.

> *and* TO OPPOSE ANY LIMIT OF CHOICES OF
> INDIVIDUALS OR FAMILIES IN REGARD TO
> FAMILY PLANNING. [Emphasis added.]

With free choice operating, as the Planned Parenthood-World Population study revealed, black birth rates are presently going down.

I consider it unconscionable from a civil-liberties viewpoint—and unworkable politically among all sections of the population—to talk of compulsory population control when so much has yet to be done to extend the exercise of free will in this matter.

In a March 28, 1972, editorial, the *Washington Post*, commenting on the report of the Commission on Population Growth and the American Future, concurred, as I do, with the commission's basic recommendations that:

> . . .(1) *States eliminate existing legal in-hibitions and restrictions on access to contraceptive information, procedures and supplies; and 2) states develop statutes affirming the desirability that all persons have ready and practicable access to contraceptive information, procedures and supplies. Indeed, the commission goes a step farther, recommending affirmative legislation which will permit minors to receive contraception and prophylactic in-*

formation and services in appropriate set-
tings sensitive to their needs and concerns.
It may be contended that this intrudes on
parental prerogatives and that it encour-
ages sexual experimentation among the
immature. Against these contentions must
be weighed the very serious hazards of
ignorance.

With regard to abortion, the commission's report
recommended that:

> *present state laws restricting abortion be*
> *liberalized along the lines of the New York*
> *State statute, such abortions to be per-*
> *formed on request of duly licensed physi-*
> *cians under conditions of medical safety.*

This agenda should be acted on immediately. And
it is my conviction that if these recommendations were
fully implemented, birth rates in this country would
continue to decline. Obviously, we won't know if this
prediction is accurate until voluntarism is given a full
chance.

Again, any attempt in the meantime to impose legal
sanctions on the individual's decisions in this area strikes
me as unconstitutional. A tax, for example, on excess
births, perhaps in the form of disallowing income-tax
deductions for more than two children, would violate not

only the doctrine of equal protection of the laws but would also directly conflict with the *Griswold v. Connecticut* decision in that people would be penalized for exercising their constitutional right to decide whether or not to have a child. Even a bounty for men willing to undergo vasectomy would be a discriminatory and, I believe, unconstitutional use of tax monies with regard to those men who do not so choose.

We have come late to the beginning of wide-scale exercise of free will concerning abortion, vasectomy, and the use of contraceptives. It is premature, let alone authoritarian, therefore, to conclude that the citizenry will not act voluntarily in its own best self-interest and that of the rest of the world. Clearly, the issue of population control is global rather than national; but, as the Club of Rome study points out,[3] the weight of responsibility for early action is on the more highly developed countries, particularly the United States. Underdeveloped countries are hardly likely to heed the warnings of the results of unbridled population growth if the wealthiest nation in the world does not first limit its own birth rate. This country is already beginning to do that and will accomplish a good deal more if there is sufficient access to birth-control information and techniques. And without government compulsion.

With the American population at its *present* level, we constitute an enormous danger to the biosphere. As

[3] *The Limits to Growth,* Donella H. Meadows et al., Universe Books, 1972.

Brian Johnson, a fellow of the Institute of Development Studies, observes: "The United States, with under 5 percent of the world's population, consumes a quarter of the world's output of fertilizer and steel, 40 percent of its wood pulp, 36 percent of its fossil fuels, and 10 percent of the output of farmland outside U. S. territory."

Even if this nation does voluntarily limit its population, we still have to recognize and act on our limits of growth, in relation to both the continued destruction of our own environment and also our grotesquely disproportionate absorption of the resources of the rest of the world.

Even with a stable, or near-stable, population, this country will have to learn to grow differently. Frank Riessman, Professor of Education Sociology at New York University, among others, has described this different kind and quality of growth:

> . . . We may be able to have enormous growth in the development of health services, education, recreation, art, culture, research, mental health, etc.—what can be called the "people services" or "human services"—while at the same time contracting industrial production, which is rapidly ripping off the resources and energy of the earth. These human-service activities are labor-intensive rather than capital and re-

> *source-intensive, and, unlike in the past,*
> *we are long on human capital and short*
> *on all other resources . . . We need a new*
> *life style which will get us away from*
> *overeating, overdriving, wasteful gadg-*
> *etry, and conspicuous consumption.*

The creation—again, voluntarily—of this new life style will require radical (getting to the root) changes in the way we educate our young and ourselves. And this, I believe, is going to be a considerably more difficult endeavor than limiting population. My suggestion to Hart Publishing Company is that another volume in this series be devoted to an exploration of how we can replace our present life style of wasteful, destructive overconsumption of "the resources and energy of the earth" with a stable, human-services state.

As a prelude to such a discussion, I reaffirm my belief in the citizenry's willingness to begin this transformation of themselves, if they are sufficiently informed of the clear and present danger to their own self-interest, and to the interests of the smaller number of progeny they are going to have—so long as this country continues to define national growth in its current terms.

The new Malthusians are performing this essential service. By specifying the catastrophic results of our present plundering of natural resources—and ecological devastation accompanying unlimited industrialization—they have started to provide the populace with the information on which we will all then have to make political decisions.

As the Club of Rome's report emphasizes:

> As soon as a society recognizes that it
> cannot maximize everything for everyone,
> it must begin to make choices.

In this country, the choice to limit population growth, I submit, is already being made; and what is needed are more means by which to enable others to decide to make that choice. We are not yet at the state, however, where enough numbers of people know viscerally, as well as intellectually, that additional limitations to growth are essential—from curbing industrialization to fundamentally altering habits of consumption. The urgent need for education now in the area of consumption goes beyond the question of product safety. Should certain products be made at all? Perhaps others should be severely limited in quantity or wholly transformed in the way in which they operate (the automobile, for example).

As a democratic socialist, I believe the majority of people will make such political decisions if they become fully informed. And in the process, they will insist on having a say as to the social consequences of what industry is allowed to continue doing.

Capitalism, even the mixed capitalism that exists in this country, is impossible to justify if life—individual life and the collective life of the biosphere—is to be sustained and regenerated. Therefore, along with voluntary population control, this country must begin to develop that human-service, socialistic society whose citizens, under political democracy, act in free will for their own best interests and those of the rest of the world.

With that addition, I agree with the Club of Rome declaration that:

> The greatest leadership will be demanded from the economically developed countries, for the first step toward such a goal [a harmonious state of global, economic, social, and ecological equilibrium] would be for them to encourage a deceleration in the growth of their own material output while, at the same time, assisting the developing nations in their efforts to advance their economies more rapidly.

We cannot expect the developing nations to advance their economies in a different way than we have unless we first take that way. And this requires more than limiting the growth of our population.

The alternative for us, individually and collectively, and for the rest of life on earth, reverberates in these lines from *Finnegans Wake:*

> Toborrow and toburrow and tobarrow! That's our crass, hairy and ever-grim life,

*till one finel howdiedow Bouncer Naster
raps on the bell with a bone and his stink-
ers stank behind him with the sceptre and
the hourglass.*

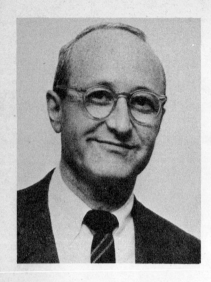

Milton Himmelfarb is the author of the new book, THE JEWS OF
MODERNITY. *He is well-known also as a contributing editor of*
COMMENTARY *magazine, for which he writes frequently, and as
editor of the* AMERICAN JEWISH YEAR BOOK.

*He was educated diversely—in the University of Paris, the City
College of New York, Columbia University, and the Jewish Theological Seminary's College of Jewish Studies.*

*Mr. Himmelfarb, who presently directs the Information and
Research Services of the American Jewish Committee, has lec-
tured at a number of universities, including Yale College and the
Jewish Theological Seminary.*

Milton
Himmelfarb

ZERO POPULATION GROWTH (ZPG) proclaims that the human population of the globe is a bomb set to explode; that the earth will soon be unable to bear the weight of a humanity multiplying exponentially, billions upon billions; that the greatest pollution of all is people pollution.

But that is more background than foreground. The foreground is the United States itself, and for ZPG the population of the United States is multiplying indecently, criminally. Soon the land area of the United States will be too small for its teeming hundreds upon hundreds of millions. Soon Americans will have no elbow room to keep themselves from psychic and indeed physical disease. Americans must start at once to decrease. They must exhort each other, or actually compel each other, to decrease.

The ZPG movement dates from the second half of the nineteen-sixties, when the rate of increase of the American population had already begun to decline steeply—so steeply, in fact, that 1,000 American women are now producing 2,110 children, the bare replacement rate. (Of course, there is no telling whether the birth rate will stay there, go up again, or drop even lower.) So, far from becoming more and more crowded, vast tracts of land have been becoming more and more empty. Anybody looking down from a plane is more apt to be struck by the emptiness of the American land than by its crowdedness.

As to what the American population problem really is, some people are beginning to worry about the bad effects of standstill and shrinkage, rather than about a nonexistent explosion. But then, such people are only sober and competent. They are not charismatic, they do not regard themselves and are not regarded by others as prophets denouncing the wicked and the selfish. Above all, they are not modish, they do not found and lead movements, they are not pronounced relevant by the media. They simply read the figures to us: for instance, that in 1970 there were 3 million fewer children under four years of age than there had been in 1960—a drop of more than 15 percent.

The interesting questions about ZPG, therefore, are not only, What is all the fuss about?—but also, Who wants the fuss? and What purposes does it serve?

Just as in the sociology of religion it can sometimes be more useful to begin by considering the laity and true believers rather than the clergy or the theologians, so with ZPG it may be more useful to begin by considering the mass rather than the elite.

As everyone knows, in the United States today, in absolute numbers and even in relative proportions, there is a constantly expanding class of young (in fact or wish), educated, progressive, critical, nonconformist individualities. This class was once described by Harold

Rosenberg as the herd of independent minds. They are like that artist in the famous *New Yorker* cartoon whose girl friend asks him, "Why must you be a nonconformist like everyone else?" For the past several years, among such people, "into" has been the favorite preposition. They have been *into* each movement and ideology that has successively been recognized as the right thing. (Who would ever have dreamt that the educated, progressive, etc., would be into I Ching, astrology, and tarot cards?) At sometime in the sixties, in that mysterious yet familiar and unmistakable fashion we all know, ZPG became the right thing to be into.

In short, faddishness—what the English call trendiness—has been at work. Yet, even fads can tell us something about the spirit of the times and people's wants. The resurgence of astrology tells us something about the irrationalism, or better the irrationality, of our day. It reminds us of something we always know but always like to forget: that rationality is a heavy burden, and that clever people easily find clever reasons for throwing off that burden.

There are two main reasons why so many clever people, especially among the modish young, have become devotees of ZPG. The first is that it is delightful to be instructed that the maximum of fun combined with the minimum of responsibility is actually moral, farsighted, and responsible. The second is that while today everybody who is anybody says he is for liberty and against arrogant technology, ZPG allows its enthusiasts—behind the screen of that ideology and without revealing to themselves what they are up to—to indulge the human, all-too-human, taste for coercion and the contemporary taste for arrogant technology. (The contradiction between a professed libertarianism and a real authoritarianism will be touched on later.)

To have children is a serious matter. It can bring joy, possibly the deepest joy available to human beings, but you can hardly say it is *fun*. It is expensive. It stands in the way of travel, skiing, dining out, theatergoing. To be a parent is to be terribly vulnerable to grief and heartbreak. It is to worry about sickness, accident, bad companions, silence. It means a lot more giving than taking—and the guilt that comes with the fear or the realization that one has not given of one's self enough. Even in these days, children assert some claim for the continuity of a marriage when, in their absence, divorce would be more convenient. Actually, without children, why marriage at all? Looser arrangements, seen as temporary from the beginning, clearly are more fun. Whatever else being a parent may be, it is not hedonism.

On the other hand, as an employee of ZPG has written, ". . . Involuntary sterilizations . . . would certainly have a liberating effect on people's sex lives." (Involuntary—i.e., compulsory, coerced; but that is for later.) If involuntary sterilization can be fun, how much more so voluntary sterilization! But not only fun; also moral, because it is responsible—responsible to the needs of a humanity, or of an American people, which,

as everyone knows, is choking to death on its own can-
cerous growth; and responsible, too, to the earth that is
being crushed under the weight of all those children,
and polluted by all that population.

That is having one's cake and eating it. One has
fun and games, taking rather than giving, and neither
vulnerability nor responsibility; and, as if that were not
enough, one is free to denounce as immorally irresponsible people who do have children.

For nobody can take seriously those declared in-
tentions to adopt children rather than beget them. For
years there have not been enough children to adopt—at
least white children. Then why shouldn't whites adopt
black children? Black intellectuals and social workers
have expressed themselves rather strongly about that,
and they are not amused. Adopt Korean or Vietnamese
children? What is that but another form of imperialism,
or of class exploitation? It means we let the natives bear
children for us—in the spirit of an aristocrat and poet of
the last century who explained, "Live? Our servants do
that for us." The very word "proletarian" comes from
proletarius, a person of the lowest class in Rome, whose
sole usefulness to society was in making *proles*, or offspring. Those who speak of adoption are trying to fool
others or themselves.

Now to the contradiction between the ZPGers'
stated horror of technology and their real love of it.
In the culture of which ZPG is part, the horror of technology is axiomatic and dogmatic. In that culture the

radicals eat macrobiotic food, and the moderates organic food; chemical fertilizers and pesticides are the enemy; technology is the enemy. We are part of nature and must live in harmony with nature. Our technology is an aggression against nature, the rape of nature. How many ZPGers would disagree?

Yet, the same people advocate, practice, and delight in the most extreme form of technological aggression—intervention into the very biology of human beings. What can be more aggressively technological than sterilization and abortion? (ZPGers insist that abortion is the only completely effective and reliable contraceptive.) And just as the mad scientist of our nightmares believes that what can be done should be done, so the abortion technologists believe that no matter how late in its life they can abort a fetus, they should abort it. And that is what their ZPG friends and supporters believe, too. Chemicals and electricity, no; reproductive surgery, sí.

For that matter, capital punishment—the ponderously legal execution of a convicted murderer—no; abortion—the private and personal killing of a living being before it emerges from the mother's womb—sí. And there are those who would not be finnicky, with respect to emergence from the womb, about the difference between before and after; between, in other words, abortion and infanticide.

The contradictions of the ZPG masses are those of the elite, though of an elite we have a right to expect something better.

In many parts of the world the population is growing too rapidly—India, China, Indonesia, Egypt, much of Latin America. Why then don't the ZPG ideologists beam their message to those parts of the world, why do they tell Americans (and Englishmen and Canadians) to stop having children? Perhaps they have tried, and find that the authorities there know well enough what the situation is, are coping in one way or another, with greater or lesser success, greater or lesser zeal, and are not especially grateful for nagging from the rich West—whose motives in any event are not assumed to be above suspicion. To justify hectoring America rather than the countries that really have a high birth rate, American ZPGers can say more or less what some American civil libertarians say when they are asked why they are more critical of the United States than, for instance, the Soviet Union, even though the state of civil liberties is infinitely worse in the Soviet Union. Let Americans criticize America and the Russians, Russia. Let American ZPGers tell America about ZPG, and Chinese ZPGers tell China.

Another way out is to say that from a global point of view, though the American birth rate may be low and the Indian birth rate high, the birth of one American baby is worse—much, much worse—than the birth of many Indian babies. In Paul Ehrlich's words, "The birth of every American child is 50 times more of a disaster"—disaster!—"for the world than the birth of each Indian child. If you take consumption of steel as a measure of overall consumption, you find that the birth of each American child is 300 times more of a disaster"—again—"than the birth of each Indonesian child." Here an American scientific intellectual is saying something very like what an American literary intellectual, Susan Sontag, has said: "The white race is the cancer of human history."

So maybe it is not too many people in general being born that the ZPG elite, or some of them, dislike primarily. Maybe what they dislike primarily is that Americans, or Westerners, are being born.

As far as I can make out, there are few demographers in the ZPG leadership. If this is so, it is curious, because about questions of the human population one would assume that it is the demographers who are expert. As far as I can make out, also, the opinion of ZPG held by the English demographer David Eversley is fairly representative of his profession. Eversley is scornful of "pseudo-scientific scaremongering and often politically motivated hysteria."

The political motivation in question is, I believe, an authoritarianism so intense that it is hardly to be distinguished from totalitarianism. This hypothesis explains why the alarm about population was sounded when the American population was *not* growing alarmingly: If you want emergency powers—authoritarian, even totalitarian powers—you must first persuade people that there is an emergency. The same sort of political motivation also explains the contradiction between the civil libertarian zeal of the academy, including the ZPG academics, and the coercion they seek for the future.

Garrett Hardin, Ehrlich's colleague in the academy and in ZPG, can speak of a maximum "X number" of children that an American woman will be allowed to have, after which she will "by law be required to have an abortion and sterilization." Conceding that "it will be a tremendous abridgment of freedom," he argues that it will be a necessary one. A ZPG colleague of his would tattoo any woman who exceeds her X number ($= 2$) of parturitions, so that all can see her infamy.

Why do people like us—educated, progressive, and so on—believe the abridgment of freedoms will be necessary then, if now, in the face of real rather than phantasmal dangers—heroin, for example, and violent crime—we deny the necessity of abridging freedoms? (That heroin is a serious danger is not the invention of reactionaries, whom all right-thinking people can immediately recognize as enemies. It is so serious that Julian Bond, no less, has urged street justice—i.e., lynch law—against pushers.) The answer given is this: The present government, or system, is wicked, corrupt, and bumbling, so we dare not entrust it with more power. On the other hand, *we* are good, honest, and able. When we ZPGers are the government, we must not be deprived of that plenitude of force we will need for setting all things right. Civil libertarian considerations were all very well in the bad old days, but now will be unnecessary, not to say harmful.

We are the true scientists. The present age's hostility to science we understand and in some measure approve, as a just retribution for the perversion of science that the old-fashioned scientists have tolerated or encouraged. *Our* science is purer and better. We are the philosophers of this age. It has always been true that the philosophers should be kings. Now the time has come when the philosophers can be kings. If the world is to be saved, we scientist-philosophers must be kings.

It is philosophers, above all, who know how to deal with the problem of quality, and the population problem is as much one of quality as of quantity. The quantity of life is too high, the quality of life too low. Lowering the quantity, we will simultaneously raise the quality. Why should diabetics, or dwarfs, be allowed birth and survival? Norman Podhoretz cites ". . . the illustrious scientist Sir Francis Crick, "who believes that no newborn infant should be declared human unless it has passed certain tests regarding its genetic endowment; if it fails these tests, it forfeits its right to live." Who will determine the conditions of forfeiture? Who but the biologists?

There are distinguished psychologists of like mind. The man regarded as the most influential psychologist in the United States calls his book *Beyond Freedom and Dignity*. He says that freedom and dignity have served their purpose and the time has come to ring down the curtain on them. His colleague, president of the American Psychological Association, calls for drugs "to subdue hostility and aggression, and, therefore, allow more humane and intelligent behavior to emerge." Who will train and direct a humanity that has passed beyond freedom and dignity? Who will find and administer those drugs? Who but the psychologists?

Between leaders and followers, between elite and mass, there is a kind of intermediate zone, in which are situated writers of letters to the editor—especially the editor of the *New York Times.* To someone "worried about abortion destroying potential geniuses," a partisan of abortion replies that "the argument might have some validity if one can prove that the fetus of today is the genius of tomorrow. But . . . we may be ridding ourselves of madmen, fools, and mediocrities, as well as Einsteins."

"Mediocrity" means "ordinary, average"—the two thirds of the population with an IQ between 90 and 110. The "fools" would then be the one sixth of the population with IQ's below 90. Between them, therefore, the mediocrities and fools who should be aborted, not allowed to live, come to five sixths of the population. Add the high-IQ madmen, and you have this educated, progressive supporter of abortion and ZPG permitting no more than 15 percent (at most) of newborn infants to live.

The writer of the letter will protest. That is not what he really means, his words are being taken with an absurd, exaggerated literalness. Very well, then, let us not hold him to literalness. Even so, he does display a jolly insouciance about those others, that large majority, who are mad, foolish, or mediocre. (I allow myself the speculation that he divides his allegiance between ZPG and Mensa.) In ZPG there is a lot of jolly insouciance about life. Maybe that is because a king is never more a king—with none of your nonsense about constitutional or limited monarchy—than when he decides, at his own pleasure and in his own judgment, who shall live and who shall die.

In a fine old movie, Ninotchka justifies Stalin's "liquidation" of millions: "There will be fewer but better Russians," she says. Under the ZPG dictators, there will be fewer but better Americans.

Since there is no American population explosion, there would seem to be no point in further discussion. But in considering some of the realities—real realities, not fake ones—that ZPG ignores, we can learn even more about its adherents and their frame of mind.

1. Americans are not all of a piece, but fall into racial, religious, ethnic, and similar groupings. (There is an embarrassment about having to write such an obvious thing, especially after the decade we have been through.) I think it was John Jay Chapman who said that while literarily and philosophically Emerson's work was infinitely superior to the typical libretto of an Italian opera, for a Martian who wanted to learn about the human race the libretto would probably be more useful

than Emerson. From the libretto he would at least learn that the human race consists of male and female. It is as if the ZPGers were Martians, unaware that Americans are white and black, Christian and Jew, Protestant and Catholic, Mayflower descendants and immigrants of various kinds.

Take a simple question: Shall the rule of two children per woman be enforced, in that fine old phrase, without regard to race, creed, color, or national origin? If the answer is yes, many thoughtful blacks will see a plot to freeze the present ratio of blacks to whites. They can argue that a racist demographic policy, governmentally enforced, would not be new in American history. After all, what was the purpose of the immigration-restriction laws of the nineteen-twenties but to freeze the ratio of non-Nordics to Nordics?

It is not that the ZPG people are anti-black. On the contrary, since the culture or ethos to which they belong ranges from liberal to radical, it is, or thinks itself, pro-black. Here we find another contradiction, between the official or conscious ideology and something less articulate, less conscious, and far more powerful—the universalist-individualist outlook, which sees only individuals, on the one hand, and universal humanity, on the other; and is impatient with the intermediate, particularist groupings of race, religion, nation.

2. The question of Jews presents a similar difficulty. If ZPG is directed against population explosion, what has it to say to the Jews, who in the past generation

have suffered a population implosion? The Jews are about 20 percent fewer now than before Hitler started murdering them in Europe. I believe that Jews should try to increase their numbers, and that the low Jewish birth rate is suicidal. An analogy can be drawn with nutrition and diet. Americans generally eat too much and weigh too much. Does that mean a physician should prescribe a reducing diet to an underweight patient? The ZPG employee I mentioned earlier will allow no exception to be made for the Jews.

3. The same sort of questions can be asked about nations and their interests. Why shouldn't the Chinese think ZPG is some kind of American or Western trick? The West is strong not in population and manpower but in machines and technique. China is strong in population. ZPG would therefore weaken China in its strength— and, because ZPG is also anti-technological, prevent China from becoming strong on the industrial side. If a country like China decides to decrease the increase of its population, it will do so for its own reasons and by a calculation of its own interests.

For ZPG, particular interests are unclean, as going against universal interests. To discourage the pursuit of particular interests, a world government—or rather a world tyranny—so crushingly powerful so as to be beyond our imagination would be needed. But would that be so bad? After all, *we* would be the philosopher-kings of that crushingly powerful world tyranny.

4. Or, again, ZPG necessarily means an aging

population, one that has a substantially higher median age than a growing population has. Some critics of ZPG do not like the prospect of a society with hardening of the arteries, condemned to old or even senile ideas, ways, and habits. I am not aware that ZPG people have answered this objection directly. It may be that privately they think the society will not be senile, because they, the philosophers, will be in charge and they will abolish senility.

For the sake of candor and as a personal afterword, I may as well set down here a few things that have influenced my views about ZPG.

1.   I came of age in the thirties, entering high school toward the beginning of the decade and graduating from college toward the end. In the thirties there was a class of people more or less like that which now heads ZPG and they, too, had firm convictions.

The most eminent American economist of the time, Alvin Hansen, knew of zero growth, but he gave it a less appealing name—"stagnation." (Has anyone noted that "zero growth" is not scientific language, but propaganda? It is language that the Ministry of Truth in *1984* might use, as it might use "zero life" for "death.") Hansen saw the stagnation in the growth of America's population as prolonging our economic stagnation, the grievous Depression. For him, and for everybody else, stagnation was not a Good Thing but a very Bad Thing. Today, right-minded people find it hard to imagine how anyone can deny the obvious truth and cogency of the zero-growth doctrine. In the thirties, right-minded people found it hard to imagine how anyone could fail to oppose stagnation.

The same applies to having or not having children. Now, the best people not only preach but also practice ZPG, and voluntary sterilization is the thing among advanced men. As I write this, I have before me an issue of the advanced *New York Review of Books*, with the following Personal:

> MALE: *Scorpio-Aries, vasectomized, separated, multifarious interests science, arts, travel. Seeks quasi-permanent liaison with stimulating good-natured youngish female. Pacific N.W.*

The same issue of the *New York Review* recommends the *Vasectomy Information Manual*.

In the thirties the best people denounced the infertility of the educated as treason to the cause of humanity. They told us that the Jukes and Kallikaks procreated like rabbits, while the average Princeton graduate had 1.3 children and the average Wellesley graduate had .7. (A favorite academic joke of statistics professors in those days: The Princeton and Wellesley data prove men have more children than women have.) Because *we* were intelligent—were we not college students?—it was our duty to improve the human stock by having more rather than fewer children. The logic seemed unassailable. If later we did not do our eugenic duty, we were apt to feel a bit guilty.

Hence my skepticism about the necessary truth of the latest truth.

2. I am a Jew, of the kind who want the Jews to continue in being, carrying forward a history of some consequence begun 3,750 years ago with Abraham. Because the Jews' being is demographically so much at risk, I want them to have more rather than fewer children.

But it does not end there. A Jewish tradition about this sort of thing is so clear that it was noted even by the pagan Tacitus in the Caesars' Rome:

> *Moses . . . gave the Jews novel religious usages . . . For the Jews everything is profane which among us is sacred . . . they think it an abomination to kill any unwanted or inconvenient child . . . The Jews understand God . . . to be one . . . supreme, eternal . . . not to be represented . . . the Jewish way is senseless and filthy.*

What the Nazis did is not ancient history—if Anne Frank were alive today, she would be forty-three years old. In conquered Holland, the Nazis offered a choice to Jewish men married to Christian women: deportation to a death camp or sterilization at home.

Three thousand years ago the Pharaoh "which knew not Joseph . . . charged all his people, saying, 'Every

[Hebrew] son that is born ye shall cast into the river. . . .'"
Two hundred and fifty years ago a Hapsburg emperor
allowed only one son of each Jewish family in Bohemia
and Moravia to marry and have children.

The scholars agree on Heinrich Himmler's "vet-
erinarian's mentality." He did not see why human
beings should be less favored than cattle, whose quantity
was controlled and whose quality was improved by
experts. Before the Nazis turned their attention to the
Jews, they were eliminating the (Aryan) diseased, aged,
deranged, and imbecile. It was only a natural, logical
next step to eliminate another inferior human element,
the Jews. For Jews, therefore, sterilization should suggest
something else than what is good for you, good for the
world, and fun besides.

Now, an illustrious scientist believes that no newborn infant should be declared human until it has passed
certain tests regarding its genetic endowment. Then, the
Jews, adult and infant, were tested by Himmler and
other geneticists like him, and found wanting. Not quali-
fying as human, the Jews forfeited the right to live.
They were murdered.

The outlook implicit in "tests regarding genetic
endowment" and "the right to live" is an abomination.

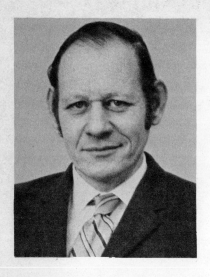

Dr. Paul Kurtz, editor of THE HUMANIST *Magazine, is a member of the Board of Directors of the American Humanist Association, the International Humanist and Ethical Union, and University Centers for Rational Alternatives. He is presently Professor of Philosophy at the State University of New York and has taught at Vassar College, The New School for Social Research, Union College, Trinity College, and many other progressive institutions.*

Dr. Kurtz has appeared as honored guest on over 150 radio and television programs, and for some time hosted his own television-interview show.

Dr. Kurtz is the author of DECISION AND THE CONDITION OF MAN, *and* MORAL PROBLEMS IN CONTEMPORARY SOCIETY; *and various other books and magazine articles on social and ethical issues.*

Paul Kurtz

THE QUESTION TODAY and in the near future is no longer *whether* there is need for a public policy regarding population control, but *when* it will occur and *how* it will be implemented. Projections of demographic growth are so overwhelming that only those totally impervious to the facts or those who are morally insensitive to their impact upon mankind can continue to ignore the situation. If present growth trends continue at the present rate, then it is likely that world population will reach 7 billion by the year 2,000, and will reach 10 billion by the year 2,020. The resultant strain on world resources, the consequent damage to the environment, and the inevitable lowering of the quality of human life would be incalculable.

Mankind seems to be fulfilling a kind of doomsday prophecy; for there are many trends accelerating at an ever-increasing tempo. In fact, the world's population may have already passed the danger point. For example, a distinguished group of British scientists and philosophers recently issued a blueprint for survival.[1] This plan contains the recommendation that Great Britain reduce her population from over 56 million in 1972 to under 32 million by the next century; for these scientists believe that she already has exceeded a healthy level.

[1] *Ecology* Magazine (January, 1972).

Throughout the world, nations are placing great emphasis on growth economics and the desire to attain larger and larger gross national products (not only in the advanced industrial nations but in the underdeveloped regions as well). If economic development elsewhere were to begin to approach the level of consumption of the United States, even if existing population levels were to remain static, the strain on world resources would be enormous. The population of the United States, though comprising less than 5 percent of the world's population, nevertheless consumes almost 40 percent of its wood pulp, one quarter of its output of steel and fertilizer, 36 percent of its fossil fuels, and 10 percent of the output of farmland outside its own territory. Any effort by the impoverished nations of the world to match America's level of affluence might spell disaster.

Although the consumption of the world's resources is expanding rapidly, these resources are finite in quantity. Fossil fuels, mineral and timber supplies, marine life, even oxygen levels, have a point of exhaustion. It is true that scientific technology and ingenuity can supplant established resources and existing technological systems with new ones, but there is no guarantee that we will be able to find substitutes for all of them. Indeed, as the pace of technological development accelerates, the uses of resources and the consequent despoliation of nature are being further aggravated.

The birth rate is a vital factor in the population

problem. More people of childbearing age are now alive
than ever before, and their numbers are constantly growing. Efforts to reduce the birth rate are succeeding in
some, if not all, parts of the world, such as the U.S.A.
and Eastern and Western Europe, but these decreases
may be too little and too late; and whether this reduced
population growth is a temporary or permanent feature
it is now difficult to say. Due to an advancing state of
medical technology, the number of fetuses and infants
who formerly died may now survive and reproduce.
Thus, population growth is still upward.

The falling death rate is another crucial factor. In
the last hundred years, life expectancy has doubled—to
seventy years or more in the advanced countries and to
fifty or more in the others. With death in childbirth reduced, infectious diseases conquered, and new drugs
and skill applied yearly, the death rate will undoubtedly
continue to drop. It is entirely within the range of probability that by the year 2,000 it will be possible to extend
the life span of large numbers of the earth's population
to one hundred, perhaps even 150 years—by improved
medical and nutritional care, by the implantation of
artificial organs, by the development of human cyborgs.
This pushing-back of death means that the question of
who shall be born will become a vital issue. Hence,
even if the birth rate were to reach zero in many other
parts of the world, this may not adequately accommodate the dislocations emerging from the increased use
of economic resources and the rapid fall of the death

rate. The problem is not simply the control of population, but the speed with which we can do so and still preserve some ecological and population balance.

Another pressing moral issue that we shall no doubt have to face is not only how to control the *quantity* of life—the number of human beings born and kept alive—but how to determine the *quality* of life, the kind of living creatures that shall be brought into being. World population control thus presents a pressing twofold problem: to limit the sheer numbers of individuals, but also to engage in some form of eugenic planning. We are rapidly approaching the time when not everyone who chooses can be permitted to bear and raise children. Shall the human race continue to depend upon blind passion, random choice, and caprice to decide who is to be born, or should we begin to adopt a conscious eugenic policy, seeking to maximize and nourish the best qualities of human life?

If we are truly able to push back the age of human death, then theoretically we may reach a point, given finite world resources, when someone can be born only when someone dies and makes a place. If bringing a new life into existence will become a relatively rarer event than it is today, then the questions of the quality of the replacement is important both for the preservation of the species and the good of human society. Society will no doubt wish to have a voice in directing and guiding the reproductive process and in selecting parents. It is an unfortunate fact that often those people who are most willing to limit their family size in order to approach zero population growth are those who are most responsible, capable, and intelligent. Conversely, it is often the poor and underdeveloped in intelligence and capacity who tend to have large families. This means that a gradual lowering of the quality of the genetic stock is likely to occur without conscious eugenic planning aimed toward improvement.

Apparently mankind has now reached the point where the very course of human evolution can and should be rationally controlled. Scientific technology has not only presented mankind with the means of restricting population growth—birth-control techniques, sterilization, abortion, etc. It now is providing us with the means, many of them startling, to determine the quality of the human life to be born—biogenetic engineering, the detection and possibly correction of genetic defects, the ability to clone individuals asexually, to reproduce in vitro, etc. We will have increasing power to choose the kinds of human characteristics that we wish to develop: intelligence, physical strength, musical ability, keen perception, and so on. Shall we do so? In controlling and restricting population, shall we also have the audacity to help create a new race of mankind? We already intervene in the course of natural selection by keeping alive those who would otherwise die and enabling them to reproduce, thus changing the course of evolution. Society is a factor in unconscious eugenics selection. Will it consciously make value judgments about the future genetic stock that we want to breed: those best adapted to a postindustrial technological and space society? This is the urgent moral challenge of the future that is pressing upon us.

One question that critics have raised is whether it is morally right to engage in massive population control and eugenic engineering. Most of the arguments seem to me to be totally inadequate to the present situation of mankind. Nevertheless, I think that they should be answered. The most familiar objections are threefold: first, religious qualms; second, moral trepidations; and third, fear that liberty of choice will be compromised. It is the third argument that I will especially examine, for there are serious reservations that many concerned persons, despite their interest in population control, raise when they realize the effect that population control may have upon individual freedom.

The religious-theological argument seems to me to no longer have any foundation. It presupposes what I consider to be an unverifiable metaphysical thesis about man and the universe. It harks back to a simpler, more peaceful state of human existence, no longer relevant to postmodern man. A doctrine of divine or natural law does have a kind of metaphysical nicety, but serious difficulties with this logic emerge when it is forced to confront the harsh realities of the real world in which we live. It is difficult to be intransigent in the face of the threatening clouds that hover over the entire human race: Such a theology flies in the face of human needs.

Nevertheless, one might say that even if God exists, human beings are not prevented from using their intelligence to control the processes of sexual reproduction, or from deciding the quality of human life that they wish to achieve. There is no necessary logical connection, as far as I can tell, between the existence of God and the practice of population control. Surely there is no empirical connection, for many men who profess belief in God nevertheless have advocated population control, including birth control, sterilization, abortion, and eugenic planning.

An influential moral objection to population control draws upon archaic phobias and commandments about human sexuality. This moral view postulates that the human individual is inviolable and that the "soul" of man ought not to be artificially tampered with. This view masks a basically Puritan attitude about sexual relations: The end of intercourse is supposedly reproduction. Yet, there are good arguments to show that physical pleasure and psychic satisfaction are basic aims of sexuality. Hence, contraception does not oppose an alleged natural function, but allows us to express love and desire without fear. The theological-moralist objection to abortion is especially saddled with a mistaken conception of human life: Is the fetus a living human personality? Surely not until it develops self-consciousness and identity. Efforts to establish human personality, or soul, at the moment of conception are contrary to the best biological and scientific evidence.

Neither the religion nor the morality of previous ages are pertinent to the present condition of the human species. Unless traditional theological and moral systems are able to reconstruct their revered values, they will suffer the charge of irrelevance. In what sense is a position "moral" if it is insensitive to the deepest human needs?

Runaway population growth will condemn billions of human beings to lives of perpetual suffering and poverty. The green revolution can only defer famine temporarily; it may not be able to do so indefinitely. Thus, population control on moral grounds seems a necessary method to achieve the greater happiness of mankind.

A powerful objection to population control, particularly for liberals and humanists, is whether the population explosion will mean an end to freedom of individual choice. Shall the state, for example, intervene in matters formerly held to be private? Shall it tell people how many children to have, when to breed, and with whom? Until now we have considered reproduction to be a matter of private choice. Will the end of this situation mean the death of liberty? The Declaration of Human Rights of the United Nations (1968) maintains that ". . . Couples have a basic human right to decide freely and responsibly on the number and spacing of their children . . ." If the state or society may now tamper with this freedom of choice, upon what grounds can it do so?

Freedom clearly is a basic moral value of libertarianism. And I would argue for a libertarian policy concerning morality. In other words, I submit that the state as far as possible ought to refrain from interfering with the tastes, desires, and values of individuals, so long as they do not harm or interfere with the rights of others. In regard to sexuality, the state ought not to tamper with the vagaries of sexual relations between consenting adults. From this point of view, laws seeking to regulate sexual morality are wrong. There should be no legal prohibitions and a minimum of regulations on abortion, adultery, homosexuality, sodomy, divorce.

Heretofore, marriage and procreation have been left to private choice. Why should we now interfere? The answer is that we may have to restrict the freedom of parenthood for the common good and the freedom of others. I wish to argue that we are reaching a situation where the only way to preserve freedom may be limitation of population. Thus, rather than argue that freedom of choice and population control are in opposition, I wish to maintain that they may go hand in hand, and that the demands of liberty require that we restrict the unlimited right of procreation (if not the right of sexuality). The state should allow consenting adults to do what they want, but only interfere if their sexual activities lead to excessive reproduction.

To say that we should be free to control our own bodies and lives does not mean that we should have the unlimited right, for example, to have five, ten, or fifteen children, without due regard for consequences to the social good. Is it impermissible for the state to say anything about my children? As a matter of fact, when there is offspring from a relationship, the state already interposes itself. One cannot bring up one's children as one sees fit without social involvement. Thus, parents may not neglect their children; they must see to it that they send their children to schools either administered, accredited, or regulated by the state; parents must properly feed their children and provide adequate medical treatment; they are not permitted to beat or abuse them. The welfare of children is considered an appropriate concern of the state. In situations of divorce, the state considers it its duty to see to it that minor children are adequately provided for. Cannot the state on the same grounds intervene in the family unit by limiting the number of children for the common good?

The arguments for interference, then, are twofold: first, to preserve individual freedom, and second, to promote the general happiness. The point is, if population is allowed to increase until it produces insufficient living space, limited resources, and undue crowding and pollution, the freedom of the individual is already seriously impaired. To increase population is to further increase the constraints on individual choice and action. In other words, random and uncontrolled population growth at some point will undermine the basic qualities of life experience for the individual: It can depress the ability to achieve a life of satisfaction, meaning, and enrichment. It will make the cherished goal of privacy impossible, as the means to achieve private goals and interests will increasingly diminish. Thus, one can argue that in the name of privacy itself, procreation can no longer be an exclusively private matter.

That we need some population control seems to be obvious. The crucial decision, however, is what methods of control we shall adopt. If one is a libertarian, one would hope that the constraints would be kept at a minimum, consonant as far as possible with a maximum of individual freedom. There exists a scale of possible means, beginning with purely voluntary efforts and ending with the use of coercive methods.

The first kinds of possible constraints are, as Malthus noted, *moral* and *rational*. They involve the use of education to awaken the public to the dangers and to inform them of safeguards that are available. Efforts to achieve zero population growth by means of public education have already had a significant impact in the U.S.A. This should become a worldwide phenomenon, entering every community and nation. If it is pursued only in the advancing nations and not in the under-developed areas, it will be inadequate. This means that there should be massive methods of persuasion, undertaken by all societies in order to develop subjective controls. It also means that there must be continued widespread education concerning the techniques of contraception, voluntary sterilization, and abortion. In addition, contraceptive devices should be made available as a free utility in high birth-rate areas (in high-school and college vending machines). Sexual education should be embarked on in the schools from the earliest grades, and there should be continuing public programs. It is encouraging, for example, that the Chinese now freely dispense contraceptive pills and the Indians encourage voluntary sterilization.

It is likewise important that new attitudes toward the family be developed. Instead of idealizing the mother with a large family, we ought to encourage late and childless marriages, even spinsterhood and celibacy. One might argue that deviant sexuality should now be viewed as a positive social good—for homosexuals do not reproduce. It is also essential that there be drastic modifications in our attitudes concerning women: Woman's place is no longer uniquely as a childbearer and in the family, but in the world as a productive citizen. Hence, we should grant full autonomy and equality to women—de-emphasizing the virtues of motherhood and emphasizing the virtues of women as full and equal partners with men.

In regard to eugenic control and therapy, society will also have to develop programs for genetic counseling of prospective parents. The medical profession should soon be able to detect possible birth defects, if possible to correct them, and if not, to abort the defective fetus. Indeed, one can conceive of gene banks where stocks of sperm and eggs are stored, and where we can choose with some degree of accuracy the kinds of children that we want to produce.

The second possible kind of constraints in population growth is *economic*. That is, the state may have to repeal all incentives to large families. Income tax deductions, family allowances, welfare, or child-care support may have to be abandoned, where they lead to larger families. There are dangers that these measures may inadvertently harm innocent children who will be penalized for the indiscretions of their parents. Hence, some means must be developed to provide adequate care for minor children; yet, at the same time the parents should not themselves be rewarded for extra children by financial bonuses.

If these measures fail to reduce fertility rates, the next step that may have to be adopted is the progressive enactment of positive de-incentives—a negative income tax, for example, whereby people who have more than two children may have to pay higher rates. For each extra child, one's taxes would increase rather than diminish. We may also have to adopt measures designed to delay marriage by charging high license fees to get married. (Much the same as it now costs several hundred dollars in lawyer and court fees to get a divorce, so it should perhaps be very expensive to get married, and there might be waiting periods as well.)

In addition to these economic measures, incentive payments may have to be made by the state to those who voluntarily restrict the size of their family. Among such incentives may be non-fertility bonuses, childless-couples-of-the-year awards, bonuses to spinsters and

bachelors, or to those who submit to voluntary sterilization.

A third set of measures, if all else fails, would be
political sanctions: We may have to limit family size by
law, to decide who can marry and reproduce, to fine
and imprison those who violate the law by producing
more than their share. In order to enhance eugenic
planning, we also may decide to prohibit reproduction
by retarded individuals or others with serious transmit-
table genetic defects. A last and desperate measure,
if all else fails, might be the reluctant resort to overt
physical coercion: the implantation of chemical aborti-
facts, mandatory sterilizations of large numbers of the
population, required abortions imposed by court order,
after due-process hearings conducted under medical
supervision.

These measures of political and physical coercion
are distasteful in the extreme. Clearly, we should as far
as possible use voluntary educational methods and rational persuasion to achieve population control. Persuasion should be our chief reliance, and there is good
hope that if pursued diligently it will prove effective.
If so, liberty of conscience will be preserved. But, if
time goes by and these methods fail, we may have to
decide upon the second set of economic measures.

We may be at that point today in many societies.
The use of political and physical coercion, however,
should be entered into reluctantly and only in desperation; that is, when there is an overriding clear and

present danger to the public good that dictates drastic measures, as in the time of an extreme national emergency or war. Prohibition, whether of alcohol or marijuana, has not been effective. It will be difficult to stamp out random sexual reproduction, and a future scenario might involve secret or covert bootlegging of babies. Yet such Draconian methods may in some instances be the only way to guarantee population control.

Liberty is a cherished value—indeed, for democratic societies, possibly the most basic value. To tamper with it is permissible only in an urgent situation. It is important that any measures of control we may institute be democratically enacted and determined only after full discussion and with safeguards. Totalitarian or authoritarian controls would be offensive. This means that corrective measures must be critically discussed and experientially entered into, always open to modification in the light of consequences and needs. Nevertheless, the most drastic measures may have to be adopted, and we should be prepared for that eventuality. No society can succeed by itself; only a world body such as the United Nations, by financial and technical assistance, can assist the backward areas to succeed.

One point is clear: Those who raise moral and theological objections to the voluntary use of contraception, sterilization and abortion, or sexual education are doing a great disservice and may be contributing to the development some day of more compulsory measures and the limitation of private choice.

It is difficult to predict with accuracy the future course of society. The contingent is always a factor in human history; unexpected eventualities such as famine or disease, a nuclear disaster, the ability to populate outer space, may alleviate population pressures on earth. History is not fixed, but depends in part upon what we do. If we can understand its trends, we can master them and not be mastered. Although passion and involuntary action play a role in human history, the real issue is whether we can transform these blind forces by means of rational control. A real test of the future existence of the race will depend on how well we respond to this challenge.

Index

Index

abortion
  as birth control, 17-18, 49-50, 62, 66-67, 90, 94, 148, 159-160, 173, 181-182, 187-188, 200, 205, 221, 226, 228-229
  in Japan, 32, 127-128
  laws, 17, 94, 148, 182, 187
  for safety of mother, 80, 81
Abraham, 211
Active Society, The (Etzioni), 157 n. 6
adoption, 62, 199
Africa, 170, 174-175
age
  at childbearing, 17, 19
  at marriage, 17, 227
  in population-growth distribution, 59-60, 89, 153-154, 208-209, 216-218
Algeria, 30
American Civil Liberties Union, 182
American Psychological Association, 205
Aragon, Manuel, 21
Armand, Louis, 117
astrology, 196
Australia, 174

"baby boom," postwar, 18-19
Baby Bust, The (Grier), 74 n. 2
Banage, William, 22
Bangladesh, 125
Berelson, Bernard, *Studies in Family Planning*, No. 38, 155 n. 4
Besant, Annie, 12
Beyond Freedom and Dignity (Skinner), 204
Bible, The, 81-82
birth control
  abortion for, 17-18, 49-50, 62, 66-67, 90, 94, 148, 159-160, 173, 181-182, 187-188, 200, 205, 221, 226, 228-229
  adoption for, 62, 199
  attitudes toward, 137-149, 155-157, 161-163, 178, 191
  availability of means for, 161, 182-183, 219, 225-226
  censorship and, 13-14
  in China, 25, 226
  coercive, 28, 31, 40-41, 49-50, 64, 78-79, 97, 99-101, 107-108, 139, 147-150, 156, 181-188, 195, 198-200, 202-203,